Praise for the *Sk*

MW00929114

Finally, a well written guidebook that gets to the root of overweight: the way people think about food.
Dr. Bernie Siegel
Author of 365 Prescriptions for the Soul

Laura Katleman-Prue's *Skinny Thinking* exposes how thought and belief can sabotage or create a healthy relationship with food and provides us with an important and empowering set of tools for transforming our relationship with how we nourish ourselves.
Georgianna Donadio, MSc, PhD
Academic Program Director
National Institute of Whole Health

FINALLY!!!! Consciousness meets food addiction. THIS BOOK IS REVOLUTIONARY! Ho, boy, am I relieved. Somebody finally wrote THE book. The book that has the possibility of truly freeing us from the bondage of food—not through another stupid diet and exercise regime, and not through another tiresome pop-psych book of feelings. What makes this book stand apart is that it goes right to the intersection of mind and mouth, where addiction kicks in, and shows you how to break that pattern with surgical precision. The strategies in this book are LIFE-CHANGING!
Lisa Holliday Lee

Skinny Thinking is an extraordinary book that guides women to a healthy weight not by providing a new fad diet, but by challenging them to permanently change their relationship with food and their bodies. Obesity is a major health problem for women and new, effective approaches are needed. Ms. Katleman-Prue teaches women how and what to eat and, more importantly, how to change the way they think about food to bring about lifelong change.
Jan L. Shifren, MD
Massachusetts General Hospital
Associate Professor of Obstetrics, Gynecology and Reproductive Biology
Harvard Medical School

My relationship with food has permanently changed! Not only am I losing weight, I know it will never come back because I look at food differently. Yea!!! I can never go back to my old ways. The steps are comprehensive and THEY WORK. I have struggled with eating and weight for years and am so delighted to have finally recovered. Your workshop and your book are the only things that have ever gotten to the root of and healed my addiction!!
Jeanne Handelman

This book provides an engaging and fun read, while offering sound advice about how thinking differently influences positive eating habits.
Gerald P. Koocher, PhD, ABPP
Dean, School of Health Sciences
Simmons College

If you truly desire to know why you overeat and want to deal with your struggles in relating to food, then this book by Laura Katleman-Prue is one you need to read.
Rev. Dr. Ed Babinsky
UCC Minister, New England Region Fitness Manager
Men's Division International

Truly unique approach to the issues of food, weight, and body image! *Skinny Thinking* is astoundingly unique, which is amazing, given the countless diet books that have been written over the past several decades. *Skinny Thinking* approaches these issues in a never-been-done-before manner by applying nondual spiritual teachings to the issues of food, weight, and body image. For me, it was the missing piece.
Susan Taft

I know I will read *Skinny Thinking* again and again, and I am sure I will keep getting more from it each time. The first few chapters were amazing. The idea of being free from the yo-yo is what really intrigued me. *Skinny Thinking* has gotten me to the place where I naturally make the right choices and DON'T THINK ABOUT FOOD! I have lost 12 lbs. since I started the book—I think it was five weeks ago—and I feel great. It is the wise eating and wise thinking that really clicked for me and have made life so much easier and stress free. I have been so excited about *Skinny Thinking* that I've been telling all my friends.
Susan Zipkin
Director, Radiology Research Finance
Brigham and Women's Hospital

Skinny Thinking is both inspirational and helpful. It gets to the root of self-sabotaging behaviors and then provides the necessary tools to heal them. Laura Katleman-Prue has done a great job of bringing us another way of thinking and acting in an age-old struggle.
Marcia Gorfinkle, RN, Life Coach/Stress Management Consultant

Skinny Thinking can change the life of any reader. Its novel approach represents a desperately needed breakthrough in this field.
Karen J. Puglia, MA, Psychotherapist

Skinny Thinking Daily Thoughts

242 Revolutionary Thoughts to Permanently Heal Your Relationship with Food, Weight, and Your Body

by Laura Katleman-Prue

ISBN: 978-1456536572
Copyright © 2011 by Laura Katleman-Prue
Published by Laura Katleman-Prue at Smashwords

This ebook is licensed for your personal enjoyment only. This ebook may not be re-sold or given away to other people. If you wouldlike to share this book with another person, please purchase an additional copy for each recipient. If you're reading this book and did not purchase it, or it was not purchased for your use only, please return it to Smashwords.com and purchase your own copy. Thank you for respecting the hard work of this author.

To Gina Lake
for your friendship, support, and guidance

FOREWORD

As Americans, we are all aware of the serious health crisis in this country. Obesity and our cultural obsession with food have reached epidemic proportions, not only among adults but among children and adolescents as well. Obesity-related illnesses result in hundreds of thousands of preventable deaths each year and billions of dollars in health care costs. As a cardiologist specializing in heart failure and transplantation, I see firsthand how body-weight issues impact my patients' health. Although my overweight patients are paying a terrible price for the way they are eating and living, the good news is that, for the most part, they can significantly improve their health by making even small changes in their dietary behavior.

Often, in spite of the best intentions, when people try to make changes to support a healthier way of living and eating, those changes are short-lived. The fact that more than 98% of the people who lose weight through dieting regain it within three years is clear evidence that focusing on diet, nutrition, and exercise alone is not enough to combat the problem. If we are to solve the epidemic of obesity, we must first concede that what we are doing is not working, and then embrace effective models of change. *Skinny Thinking Freedom Thoughts* is a distillation of all of the important concepts in the original *Skinny Thinking* book, provides such a model.

Skinny Thinking is a remarkable compendium of tools and information that guide readers to a healthy body weight not by providing a new fad diet, but by challenging them to permanently change their relationship with food, their thinking, and their bodies. Ms. Katleman-Prue teaches people who have issues with food and body weight not only how and what to eat, but, more importantly, how to alter the way they *think* about the food they eat to bring about lifelong change.

The American health care system is failing to solve the growing pattern of obesity and other chronic conditions. The situation can only be solved by changing our health care paradigm from illness to wellness. To this end, I have begun to shift my practice toward disease prevention and self-directed wellness. I'm convinced that, ultimately, the way to achieve wellness and prevent disease is through exploring the connection between mind, body, and spirit. Among other things, I've seen the enormous impact of patients' habitual thinking patterns on their prognosis for healing once they've suffered a serious illness.

Similarly, I have no doubt that those who suffer from eating and body-weight issues engage in habitual thinking patterns that sabotage their healing efforts. This is precisely why I am excited to endorse *Skinny Thinking*. Not only is it the first book to address the role our thoughts play in health issues, it also identifies "romantic thinking" about food as the core problem. But this insightful book doesn't stop there. Because food and eating issues are complex and multifaceted, touching every aspect of life, solving them requires a whole-person approach. The *Skinny Thinking* Five Steps encompass everything from food choices, lifestyle, and eating habits, to basic emotional well-being, questioning misguided beliefs about food, and learning to connect and align with the spiritual dimension of being.

If you suffer from eating or body-weight issues and are ready to stop the cycle of yo-yo dieting, the book you now hold in your hands will provide the tools and insights you need to succeed. Just follow the simple Five Steps. My advice to every

SKINNY THINKING
DAILY THOUGHTS

1.

There's a way of thinking about food that's a problem, and a way of thinking about it that isn't a problem, and the problematic way corresponds to feeling out of control around food and to having a heavier body. Your *relationship with food*, which is based on how you think about it, makes all the difference. You have different relationships with your mother, your brother, your friend, your boss, and your lover, and you think about all of those people differently. In the same way, you have an easy or challenging relationship with food, depending on the way you habitually think about it.

2.

How do you relate to food? As a lover, a friend, a god, an enemy, a source of nutrition? What is your image of yourself in relationship to food? What are the thoughts and self-images that mediate between you and food? When you remove all of the thoughts and images that mediate between you and food, what's left? Just a simple, pragmatic relationship with food.

3.

Set the intention to develop a simple, pragmatic relationship with food. This means learning to align with your true nature rather than with the false self or ego. When you are in touch with what I call *the true self* or *the Wise Witness*, you are in touch with a mature, wise part of you at the core of your being. When you are aligned with that, rather than with the ego or negative thoughts that constantly chatter in your head, you feel happy and at peace.

4.

The ego experiences separation from other people and creates the fear at the root of your suffering, including your eating-related suffering. When you are identified with the ego instead of the Wise Witness, you innocently make choices that are contrary to your physical, psychological, and spiritual well-being. You relate to food from your conditioning, and this causes you to look for things from food that it cannot provide. When you are aligned with the ego, you may overeat or eat the wrong foods because your uninvestigated thoughts are mediating between food and you. The ego tempts you with a thin sliver of truth, the pleasurable aspect of eating, and filters out everything else. Then, based on this slant, it creates desires and drives that interfere with a simple and natural relationship with food. Those desires and drives impel you to reach for food whether you're hungry or not, and before you know it, the pounds are piling on.

5.

When you're able to drop out of the ego and move into alignment with the Wise Witness, you're able to see a pure, practical way of eating that's based on food's true function. This includes it nutritional value as well as the taste pleasure it provides. The Wise Witness's way of relating to food includes the entire picture—"the whole truth about food."

12.

Be kind with yourself about having a food issue. Look around you. Most people have challenging relationships with food. In the case of food and weight, our egoic mind pits two stubborn, mutually exclusive desires against each other: the desire to experience taste pleasure from food and the desire look good. No wonder we're in a pickle! On the one hand, our bodies need food to survive and we're programmed to adore food. On the other hand, we're bombarded with media images of young, thin, attractive people and brainwashed into thinking that we should look that way, too.

13.

Never chastise yourself for having a food issue. The good news is that the food and weight issues that have been the bane of your existence are also your custom-designed ticket to freedom.

14.

Healing means:

Permanently changing your diet. Changing your diet means changing what you're eating habitually so that most of your calories come from healthy, nutritious, whole foods, and eating those foods in reasonable portions.

Changing your relationship to food by changing the way you habitually think about it. Bad eating habits in part stem from the way you've been thinking about food.

A bird needs both of its wings to fly, and healing your food issues requires both of these two components to be complete and lasting—a shift in your diet and a change in your relationship with food.

15.

The only reasonable diet to ever go on is a "thought diet," questioning and debunking the fantasies that have been mediating between you and food.

16.

Self-inquiry is a crucial part of healing eating and weight issues. It's a truth-telling tool to bust through your illusions and beliefs about food. Ultimately, you must begin to let go of deluded, misguided beliefs and your romanticized relationship with food in order to stop suffering and yo-yoing. In my experience, the best tool to achieve this is inquiry.

17.

The truth can't be changed, because the truth is always the truth. You can't continue to eat the way you've been eating and have the healthy body you want. It's simple and unambiguous. Yet many of us have been in denial, pretending that it isn't so. We want to look good, feel good, and keep eating all the junk we want. C'est impossible!

18.

It's natural to look for a way to somehow have your cake and eat it, too, to somehow maintain your bad habits, and still enjoy a healthy, slim body. It seems like other people can do it, right? Why not you? But do you really know what other people are doing to maintain thin bodies while they scarf down massive slabs of chocolate fudge cake? Very few people can eat whatever they want and stay thin. Even if they manage to stay thin, what are the health consequences of eating all that junk? Once again, the truth is still the truth: You have to change your old habits if you want to heal this issue. Only then will you start to reap the rewards.

19.

If you trade your old eating and thinking habits for healthy ones, over time you will naturally settle into a healthy weight. Rather than focusing on a goal weight, as you might have done when you were dieting, focus on not going back to your old habits. You might as well just bite the bullet. Look yourself squarely in the eyes and tell yourself the truth: "_____, you can never go back to your old habits and stay thin." This is the truth that most people don't want to face.

20.

To be really free, you have to transform your relationship to food forever. You have to be willing to change the way you eat and think about food and never go back. That's the simple, kind truth of it. Now go forth and heal! You can do this!

21.

If, like many people, you find yourself eating when you're not hungry, it's likely that you're using food to get happy, and you can learn to change that habit. Remember to ask yourself if you are hungry before you eat today. Eating when you're not hungry creates a cycle of suffering: You eat to get happy, feel bad for indulging, and then eat more to escape your emotional discomfort.

22.

Don't feel bad for having body and eating issues. They can actually help us see our way to a happier life once we realize that the way we've been thinking and living doesn't serve us. The stressful issues that dog us year after year are most instrumental in catalyzing our growth. Even though they hurt like heck, they're ultimately our ticket to freedom from suffering. Suffering moves us to break free from our unconscious patterns and conditioning and instead live from the true self. In this state, we are free to experience the peace and joy available in each moment. This is the battle: resistance versus acceptance; the ego versus the true self; self-delusion versus truth; the ego's small sliver of truth about food and the body versus the whole picture.

23.

The Critic is the judgmental voice inside our head berating the way our body looks, telling us, "You're too fat."; "Your chest is too small."; "Your thighs are too big."; "You need to look like the images you see in the media—young, thin, and beautiful."; and "You'll never attract the kind of relationship you want unless you get into better shape." When it comes to food, the pleasure-seeking Child causes us to gain weight by telling us things like "You've been working so hard, you deserve a slice…or two…or three of cheesecake."; "You should live a little. Give yourself a treat."; "Eating a bit more won't hurt."; "You've had a lousy day, so why not make yourself feel better with a little pleasure food?"; and "Indulge now and worry about tomorrow tomorrow." The Child creates our eating problem by tempting us to use pleasure food as a treat, cajoling us to eat a few more bites even when our stomachs are bursting. Then, the Critic has the unmitigated gall to shame and castigate us over the weight gain the Child caused!

24.

Don't let yourself fall for the Dreamer's entreaties. When we're upset because we've eaten too much or eaten the wrong foods, the ego in the form of the Dreamer rides in on a white steed, offering salvation—a new diet that will rid us of our excess weight and let us become the sexy vixens we've always known we could be.

25.

The more time we spend in the true self, the easier it is to heal our eating issues and lose weight. The Wise Witness *is* our true self, the one who naturally knows what to eat to keep us healthy. It's who we are when we're not listening to and believing in the ego. It's that inner place of calm and serenity that we've all visited in moments when the mind is quiet. Think back to a time when you've felt completely at peace. That delicious feeling is the true self. Even though we may not be aware of this consciously, each of us taps into it every day! Make it a point to connect with your true self, right now! Move out of the thinking mind into the stillness of your true self by asking yourself, "Where's the quiet?" If you want to experience life from a delightful place of openness, wonder, and curiosity, you have to relearn how to connect with the true self, shedding what no longer serves you so that our natural state of radiant happiness shines through.

26.

Connecting with the Wise Witness means entering the thought-free state beyond identification with our minds and bodies. Although meditation is the most common way to move out of the mind, we can do this anywhere, anytime, <u>as long as we're not caught up in thoughts or feelings.</u> We can notice the clock on the wall, a leaf floating in the breeze, or our hand as we turn the page. Information from the senses, before thought comes in, takes us to the true self. If we are to break the habit of paying attention to and following our thinking, which is responsible for our food issues, it helps to cultivate a new habit of diving into the space between our thoughts. Spend at least 10 to 15 minutes today sitting quietly, either in silence or while listening to restful music. And then do the same thing tomorrow, the next day, and so on!

27.

Notice the place you are eating from today. There are two ways to approach eating: from the Child's point of view (our conditioning, which is part of the ego), or from the true self's point of view. Whenever we're eating to fill a psychological need rather than a physical need, we're identifying with our conditioning. The true self, on the other hand, encourages actions that support the optimal functioning of the body, so it's unlikely that the true self will move us to overeat when we've had enough.

28.

Don't be fooled by the ego today! The ego seduces us into eating too much of the wrong foods, and then berates us afterwards. Anything to control us! Luckily, just because it is trying to tempt us doesn't mean we have to pay attention to it. You are in control of your attention. If you don't like what's playing on ego radio, simply turn it off. When you notice that you're eating to fill a psychological need, simply being aware of it can shift you back into the true self. *When you're able to notice your conditioning, you stop identifying with the ego and start identifying with the true self.* It's that simple. Noticing it is all it takes.

29.

Today, rather than following the well-worn path of emotional eating, set the intention *not* to do that. You can ask yourself, "Is this really what I want to be doing right now? Will it satisfy me forever?" This moves you out of identification with your conditioning and into the true self, your own inner wisdom. Eat from the true self today. You can tell you're in the ego is when you're eating without any conscious connection to the food or the body. You eat unconsciously when you're either caught up in thought or in the midst of an emotional upset. Neither is a good time to eat because you can't pay attention to how full you're getting. Before you know it, you're stuffed and you haven't fully experienced or enjoyed the experience of eating.

30.

The ego is the voice of the extreme. On one hand, it advocates excess and indulgence and on the other, rigid restriction or deprivation. Whenever eating results in suffering, we know we're in the ego. Listen for the messages that come to you from your true self today. It always advocates balance, health, and temperance. It's quiet and doesn't fight for your attention, but nudges you and speaks to you through our intuition. For example, if you're grocery shopping, you may feel moved to buy something healthy that wasn't on your shopping list. This subtle nudging is from the true self, moving you in a direction that serves the body's well-being.

31.

Today bring more awareness to your eating. Are you aligned with the ego or the true self when you pick up a fork? Are you engrossed in thought or are you present, experiencing directly whatever is happening now? To align with the true self, continually bring your attention back to *awareness* by asking yourself, "What's happening in this moment?"

32.

Dating back to childhood, you may have been overeating to get happy and stuff uncomfortable feelings. This may have been how you loved yourself. Now close your eyes and take a moment to really see that this way of caring for yourself doesn't serve you and creates suffering rather than happiness and comfort. What does food mean to you? Live in this question. What is the emotional connection you've created with food?

33.

Make it a point today to really be present when you are eating. Ironically, those of us who love food and see it as central to our happiness are not very aware when we're eating. We find ourselves eating quickly or while doing something else, such as driving, talking on the phone, watching television, or reading, so the experience of eating isn't as satisfying as it could be.

34.

Today ask yourself these questions, "When and why am I deciding to eat something? What are my eating triggers? How am I feeling while I'm eating?" Notice if you are present in the experience of eating, or is your mind somewhere else, engaging in problem solving or ruminating over a frustrating experience. What are the emotions and thoughts that send you racing toward the fridge? When you're bored, is your first impulse to get some food?

35.

Today become aware of portion size. Notice how much food you're putting on your plate. Is it a reasonable amount? Many of us are used to eating portions that are much larger than we need.

36.

Today, be aware of your other eating activities. What else are you doing when you're eating? Are you driving, surfing the Internet, watching television, or having a heated discussion?

37.

Thoughts lead to feelings and feelings lead to actions. The way you think about food creates certain feelings and those feelings lead to eating. You can force off weight by going on a diet, but just like when you pull off the top of a weed, the problem will come right back if you don't take care of the root. A thought about food is just a thought, like any other. In and of themselves, thoughts have no power. I repeat, *thoughts have no power*—none, nada, zilch! The ego wants you to believe that you can't ignore a food thought and that you have to follow it, that once a food thought is on the scene, you have to find and consume pleasure food right away. But that is just the Child lying to you. Today, if you're thinking about food when you aren't hungry, ask yourself, "What experience am I trying to avoid right now?"

38.

The key to healing is becoming more aware of how you think about food and how often you think about it. The problem with thinking about food is that it leads to eating. Of course, this isn't a problem if you're actually hungry and it's time to eat. But if you're in the habit of thinking about food often, it's likely that you're eating more food, and more pleasure food in particular, than your body needs. Thinking about food can become our mind's default position, coming in whenever we are stressed, excited, overwhelmed, upset, elated, or bored—any excuse to think about food will do.

39.

Close your eyes and imagine overeating a pleasure food when you're not hungry. What are the costs and benefits of this choice? The Child tempts you by getting you to fantasize about tasting something delicious. But it doesn't tell you about the negative consequences of indulging a pleasure food craving when you're already full.

40.

Overeating when your stomach is full requires a degree of self-delusion. In these moments, the Child is in charge because you're considering only taste, not health. You're thinking, "This tastes really nice. I want more of it, even though I'm full." To keep eating when you're full, you have to put blinders on and be willing to see only part of the truth, be willing to say to yourself, "Right now, I'm more interested in immediate gratification than any negative longer-term consequences." The next time the Child comes on the scene, you can counter her pleadings with a mental image of this table. You can then say, "Hold on a minute. You're not telling me the whole truth, that in exchange for spending a few short seconds with a pleasure food, I'll suffer for hours, days, or even weeks. That's a lousy trade-off. It's not worth it."

41.

But how do you break the habit of turning to food in your time of need or celebration or longing? The answer is: Take another look. Open yourself to a broader perspective and come to see the whole truth about food rather than just hanging on to your habitual, unquestioned assumptions. In your moment of wanting a pleasure food, nothing seems clearer or more powerful than your desire. In those moments, the Child is powerful; she has your undivided attention and it takes tremendous will to say "Not now, dear, maybe later," just as you might to a child who wants a snack right before dinner. Listening to and following the dictates of the Child is a habit that has grown stronger through years of repetition and reinforcement. But if you believe that breaking this habit is daunting, just remember—you created it in the first place, so you have the power to uncreate it.

42.

Of course, the ego wants you to view the desire to experience the taste pleasure of food as impossible to resist because that keeps you from challenging the ego's authority. But now is the time to let go of this false story that you've created. Realize that you are kingmaker and you have the power to debunk your story and withdraw your misguided projections about food. The power of choice has always rested in you. Dethrone food by changing the way you think about. It's just nice tasting nutrition, not your lover, your friend, your main source of comfort or life's greatest pleasure.

43.

If the Child is tempting you with pleasure food and you're not hungry, ask yourself: "What am I telling myself that's creating the impulse to reach for food? What am I thinking? What am I feeling right now?" Then ask yourself if eating the pleasure food will truly satisfy that impulse. Will it alleviate the feeling? Will it solve the problem that you're ruminating over? Will it rewrite history or alleviate worries about the future? Will it allow you to say the things you wanted to say in that conversation with your coworker or spouse or child? What will two minutes with that particular food give you? Are the negative consequences of shame, blame, self-castigation, lethargy, ill health, and weight gain worth it?

44.

Once you've seen the whole truth about food, you can't believe in it or idolize it in the same way. This inexorably changes you and sets the stage for a new, pragmatic, rational relationship with food. See food for what it always has been—not a god—just food with a lowercase "f."

45.

If you notice an urge to eat something when you're not hungry, you're probably involved in a story—something negative that the mind is telling you about yourself, life, others, or something you're doing. At those moments, you're arguing with reality, resisting the way life is showing up. The habit of eating pleasure food to change your experience, to escape and entertain yourself rather than nourish your body, is an innocent way of trying to love and soothe yourself when your bored or under stress. There's no reason to make yourself feel bad or wrong about this. However, overfilling your tank has consequences that don't feel loving, like indigestion, lethargy, or feeling bloated, nauseated, headachy, or sleepy. You may feel guilty, regretful, or angry, and judge yourself for lacking willpower when you gain weight and your clothes feel tight.

46.

If you notice your hand reaching toward the cookie jar or the ice cream in the freezer when you're full, walk into another room, away from the food and ask, "What story am I in?" or "What am I believing that's not true?" or "What do I really need right now?" Get quiet and take a few minutes with these questions. Almost always, you will find a painful emotion or some unease lurking underneath this impulse.

47.

One of the costs of overindulging in pleasure food is that it prevents you from experiencing or inquiring about what you're feeling or believing that caused you to want to eat. The Child goes after pleasure as a way of coping with what it doesn't like about life. When you automatically indulge and fulfill a desire, you miss out on its real message: There's something that's off here that I need to address, either inside myself, in my life, or with another person. Keep this in mind and notice when the Child starts talking to you. Ask yourself, "Is there something that I'm resisting about life, something that I'm trying to cope with by seeking pleasure? Why do I need pleasure now? What do I really need?" If you uncover a belief or story that causes you to feel bad and overeat, like a good prosecutor, begin to gather evidence to support the veracity of your belief. Is the story you're telling yourself true? If you're going to believe something and let it ruin your mood and run your life, shouldn't it at least be true? As a reasonable, rational person, shouldn't that be your minimum requirement?

When you are tied up in a negative story, ask yourself, "Can I absolutely know that this is true? Can I know that I shouldn't have to do this task? Is it really true that I'm always making a mess of things or that so-and-so is always busting my chops?" Beliefs that cause you to suffer are big fat lies or, at the very least, partial truths.

48.

Beliefs that cause you to overeat and feel bad only contain a sliver of truth, but that the ego used that sliver to hook you. Thankfully, when you see that you've been suckered—really see it—you become liberated from those beliefs. If they arise again, you can notice them, and flick them away like you would a mosquito.

49.

Slow down and notice what happens during a meal. When you first sit down, assuming you're hungry, the first few bites taste delicious. But as you move toward satiation, the experience changes, the law of diminishing returns sets in, and each successive bite becomes less pleasurable. Once you're satiated, the pleasure drops off even faster, until each additional bite becomes downright unpleasant!

50.

Eating pleasure food has a tendency to turn into overeating pleasure food. One of the characteristics of pleasure food is that it tastes so darn good that it's hard to stop eating it. How can you be expected to resist eating more of something that was designed to be irresistible? Even when you're stuffed and your stomach is groaning, you still want to taste more. You delude yourself into thinking that if you continue eating, you can squeeze a bit more pleasure out of the experience, but alas, all you get is pain.

51.

The human impulse to hold on to pleasure and avoid pain is an important part of the whole picture of food. Desire is governed by duality, and overindulging in pleasure is inexorably linked to pain. Just like trying to separate two sides of a coin, you can't peel the pleasure away from the pain.

52.

Food tantalizes our senses, beckoning us with mouthwatering aromas and titillating tastes and textures. Compounded by the fact that, as human beings, we're programmed to love food, we have a perfect storm for an overeating and weight-control disaster. Eating is pleasurable, and there's nothing wrong with enjoying food. Yet when food becomes the object of your desire, your secret passion, entertainment, or a naughty indulgence, you've turned it into something it's not—a lover.

53.

Unconsciously, we can imbue food with the power to fill many physical and emotional needs. But it was never designed to do that. Ultimately, healing means withdrawing our romantic projections, seeing food as nice-tasting nutrition, not the stuff that we can't wait to curl up with and get into our mouths. Rather than, "Oh, sweet brownie, how I love you and long to taste your rich, chocolaty goodness," our food thoughts might sound like, "I'm hungry and it's time to eat. What will I have? My body could use some protein and vegetables. I have X in the house, so I will create Y meal." Although it may not be sexy or exciting, this new way of thinking sets the stage for a healthy, rational, mature relationship with food.

54.

If you eat for pleasure, chances are that you see food as your friend, a treat, or a reward rather than just as nourishment. It's a very deeply embedded view in which food becomes larger than life, taking on a glorified and revered position in your life. You blow its importance out of proportion relative to what it can actually offer you. Because you see your relationship with pleasure food as more important to your happiness than it truly is, if you allow yourself to eat it after abstaining from it on a diet, you can easily go hog wild.

55.

\The pleasure from eating is fleeting! Soon after you put something in your mouth, the experience of eating is over. That's part of the whole truth that the Child doesn't want you to know. It's liberating to realize that if you don't have two minutes with a particular food, it really won't impact your life.

56.

When we habitually think about food in a way that creates excitement and pleasurable sensations, it makes food seem wonderfully fun and special, and this can leave us in an emotionally charged trance of sorts. Without realizing it, we slip into another state of consciousness, where seeing the whole truth about food is impossible. Once we realize how untrue and overblown our thinking is about it, we're well on our way to thinking about it differently.

57.

Glorifying food is a habit of believing that we need it to be happy and to feel good. But we don't. As we examine our beliefs about food and discover the truth, we realize that we never needed to get pleasure from food because life itself is pleasurable.

58.

The truth about loving food is that at a certain point, it stops loving you back. Actually, that isn't even true. Food can't love you back. Food is just food. It's fuel that gives the body energy to go about its business. But it's fuel that tastes good and is pleasurable to eat, and that's an undeniable part of the eating equation.

59.

With so many other pleasures available, why have so many of us become fixated on and addicted to food? What's its allure? I'd wager that most would say that food captures our hearts and imaginations because it looks, smells, and tastes so good. It activates all five of our senses. From the moment that we lift food-laden forks to our lips, there is no denying the pleasure it gives us. Or is there? Are we totally sure about this pleasure assumption? Image eating your favorite food all by yourself with no other distractions. Does this sound appealing? If not, why not? If food were truly the love of your life, why would you need to couple eating with other activities? Why isn't eating, this so-called most pleasurable experience, enough? Hmm? Maybe, just maybe, your idea of eating doesn't match up to the truth about it. Maybe you haven't been seeing the whole truth about food.

60.

There is no denying that while food is in our mouths, it tastes good. Yet prolonging the pleasure means inserting more and more food. And if we do this, we all know what happens. When we follow one bite with another and end up overfilling our stomachs, in no time, the experience of eating shifts into something else. The pleasure turns into pain. The excited anticipation turns into aversion. The truth about loving food is that it tastes good for only a short while and if we try to draw out its taste pleasure, our love soon turns to hate, and weight gain, guilt, self-castigation, lethargy, and aversion follow in quick succession. Does it really make sense to romanticize an experience when the pleasure you derive from it is so fleeting? Or are there other ways you can take care of yourself that are *truly* fulfilling and nurturing? Ask yourself, "How can I feed my soul and experience the kind of joy that can't fade or turn into its opposite?"

61.

An important part of withdrawing your romanticization of food is finding other activities that are pleasurable and meaningful, other than food. What are other "10's" for you? What do you enjoy that doesn't bring the suffering that accompanies your all-consuming love affair with food? Food may never become a "1" for you, but hopefully, after practicing the Five Steps, you will be able to see it as a "5" or a "6."

62.

Healing our food issues means that we learn to stop glamorizing food by withdrawing some of our false projections onto it and false meanings we've given to it. A balanced relationship with food would be more like your relationship with toilet paper. Okay, I admit this is a crude analogy, but with both food and toilet paper, quality is important. They both fill a need (when you need it, you need it!), the experience of using them is quick, and most importantly, there's no need to think about them when you're not using them. It's not like you're going to create an overblown fantasy anticipating the velvety softness of two-ply Cottonelle!

63.

Take a moment now to notice any romantic thoughts you might have about food and ask if these projections are really true. Can food fulfill you and give you lasting pleasure? When you go without food and don't think about it, you see the truth: You really don't need food as a source of pleasure. Of course, you need it to survive, but you don't need to have a certain food at a particular time. When you don't think about food, you're free of it, and you see that you don't need to have a romance with it. Then, your relationship with it can become very practical and healthy. Instead of dreaming about food like you might fantasize about sex, notice the pleasure in being alive, in performing simple everyday tasks, and in thinking about food in a practical way. The romantic relationship with food disappears as you see the complete truth about what it can and can't offer you. The way we think about food is the crux of our problems with it. If your romanticism of and longing for food go away, then your problem with food goes away.

Feelings manifest as sensations in the body, making them seem much more real than thoughts. If we feel a certain way, that feeling must be true, right? As if this weren't enough, inflated by self-righteousness, the ego comes up with all the reasons why *we're right* about our feelings, feeding a given emotion with more thoughts, pumping it up until it achieves its desired objective—action. The ego is always looking for a fight, and the worse we feel, the better it likes it.

64.

Feelings come from thoughts. It seems like this should be common knowledge, found in a standard-issue operating manual on how to live as a human being. Just think—if we had known that feelings come from thoughts when we were children, we could have learned to deal with our stressful thoughts by either ignoring or questioning them. In fact, we could have avoided creating negative feelings in the first place!

65.

Maintaining our emotional hygiene by debunking negative thoughts can become second nature—the only sane way to live. We have the power to stop creating negative emotions. When a stressful belief arises, we can catch it and say to ourselves, "Oh, that's just conditioning." and ignore it. If we buy into a belief and accidentally created a negative feeling, we can ask, "What am I believing right now that's causing me to feel this way?" That question can yank us out of the ego and transport us back to the rational, pleasant world of the true self.

66.

We have become accustomed to listening to and believing stressful thoughts that create anger, sadness, and fear. With practice, though, we can learn to catch feelings before they form. We can form a new habit of ignoring the egoic mind and seeing thoughts as simply results of our conditioning.

67.

One reason our feelings feel so real and overwhelming is that we identify or merge with them. We become the anger or sadness or fear. We think that it's *our* anger and feel self-righteous about it: "It's mine, and I have a right to express it, and you'd better respect it! But who says that feelings belong to us? Or even that thoughts belong to us? Both arise and subside unbidden. If we feel ownership of our emotions and believe they're meaningful, it will be harder to let them arise and subside naturally. We'll want to hold on to them, feel their power, and feed them with more thoughts and beliefs that justify their presence. Then, we'll want others to validate our position and our right to feel what we feel.

68.

Remember that you are *that which is aware* of emotion, rather than the emotion itself, it will have far less power over you. From this vantage point, you can watch the action without getting involved in it. For example, anger happens. It arises, it's felt, it does its dance, it subsides—and you remain unchanged. You are only the space in which anger arises and are completely unsullied by it.

69.

Anger is the Critic saying to life, "Oh, no you didn't." Stress is how we put a nice face on anger. It's anger in disguise. It's the ego getting mad at life, God, and whoever else is around, saying, "This is too much. Life feels overwhelming. I don't have enough time or energy to do all of this!" anything that will get me out of there. Of course, the Child has an easy answer—reach for something yummy to eat.

70.

Whenever we're upset about what's happening, we're arguing with reality. Life in the form of a particular situation has already happened. It's a fact, and there's nothing we can do about it. As author Byron Katie says, "When we fight with life we lose, but only 100% of the time!" Our resistance to life is created by the thought "This shouldn't be happening." This is the most common way that we cause our own suffering. Whenever we're irritated by a situation—we're waiting in a traffic jam or someone breaks a promise—the mind tends to jump in and proclaim that this or that *should* be different: "There *should* be more staff on the cash registers so that people don't have to wait for such a long time." "They *shouldn't* make a promise they can't keep." "They *should* have known better." "This slow car in front of me *should* go faster."

71.

Notice what happens when you use the word "should." There's an immediate contraction in your body. You're resisting life and that doesn't feel good. Your perspective narrows down to a tiny sliver of the truth about a situation and you miss seeing the whole picture. Seeing only the reasons why things *should* be different, you don't consider the possible benefits of the situation. Today, if you're standing in a long checkout line at the supermarket or stuck in traffic, consider the possibility that waiting provides an opportunity for quiet contemplation. If someone lets you down or breaks a promise, it gives you a chance to learn tolerance or discernment: Remember how it felt when you made a promise that you didn't keep or let someone down, and sidestep judgment and learn compassion and forgiveness, instead.

72.

Today if something happens that you don't like, look at the potential benefit that comes with this new development. You don't have to jump right to the downside or what you think should be happening, as you might have done in the past. Considering the benefit eliminates the reaction altogether. Don't be discouraged if it takes a lot of practice to get to this point.

73.

If you notice anger arising today, you can recognize that your conditioning is coming up in the form of anger and say, "Oh, that's just my conditioning." This noticing helps you dis-identify with your negative story and let it go. If you're quick enough, you'll notice and dis-identify with it before the anger or stress has a chance to erupt in your body! If you get triggered today, acknowledge it. You can say something like, "Wow, I've really been triggered," or "I'm really in reaction." Noticing and telling yourself the truth brings you back to the present moment, takes you out of the story you're running and into the Wise Witness. *Be gentle with yourself and let it be okay that you're in reaction.* Ironically, this will move you into acceptance! Once you're in acceptance, even if you found it by accepting the fact that you're in resistance, you can go back to your true self!

74.

We've come to believe that when the Child comes on the scene, we have no choice but to listen and follow her directions. The truth, though, is that the past is *not* a reliable predictor of the future. Just because you've reached for food 620,000 times before doesn't mean you have to do it now. You can choose health over your conditioning, your true self over the ego. Rather than listening to the Child coaxing you down a self-destructive road to food hell, ask yourself if you're willing to try something different. Just this once, are you willing to stop the action and not reach for food?

75.

Instead of stuffing down the depression or sadness with food, could you allow it to be present and ask yourself, "What story am I in right now? What am I believing that's causing me to feel flattened and down on myself and life?" You can even tell the Child that she can still eat later, if that's what she wants, but not right now. The next time depression or sadness is on the scene, try this experiment and see what happens.

76.

When we're bored, we tell ourselves the unhappy story that whatever is happening is uninteresting and not what we were hoping for from life. We feel restless and dissatisfied. Oftentimes, when we tell ourselves a story that results in boredom, we move into default mode—reaching for something tasty. We allow the Child to take over, and see food solely as a source of pleasure. One way to avoid reaching for food when boredom strikes is to say to the Child, just as we might to a persistent two-year-old, "Not now—maybe later." The Wise Witness remembers the "whole truth about pleasure food," that even though it may taste nice for a few fleeting seconds, it can't alleviate boredom. If we eat it and we're not hungry, it may not taste as good as we had imagined or we may overeat it and end up feeling worse because we gave into our craving. Seeing the whole truth about food from the perspective of the Wise Witness, interrupts the automatic tendency to reach for food when we're bored.

77.

If you eat to numb out, you miss the opportunity to heal whatever conditioning is arising. The next time you're bored, ask yourself "What is my true self's experience of boredom?" You know the ego's experience, but become aware of how your true self *just notices* the boredom. It isn't the generator of the feeling (the ego is), and it isn't affected by it either. It just notices boredom arising and doesn't evaluate it as something to like or not like. It isn't trying to get life to conform to a certain feeling. It's just humming along, okay with everything as it is. When boredom arises, you can become aware of it and realize that it's not who you really are. In other words, you can dis-identify with it. Who you are is able to notice the ego being bored. Simply allow the feeling of boredom to be present and reengage in what you're doing. When you allow a negative feeling to be present without trying to make it to dissipate or when you're fully engaged in what you're doing, you're not thinking. And if you're not thinking, you automatically align with your true self and you can't be bored. What a blessing!

78.

At their core, fear and worry are about survival. The egoic mind invents a scary future and you're instantly trapped in fear's clutches. 90% of the things you fear wil never happen. Just because fear and worry arise doesn't mean you have to avoid them through food. They can't hurt you and like all other feelings, they eventually dissipate. You can allow them to be present and learn to tolerate them after all. The best way to deal with fear and worry is to ask, "What's the worst thing that could happen?" Then you see that even if the worst thing happens, you can deal with it and then, fear lets go of you and you can rest.

79.

One important step in dealing with feelings is to *slow down the action*. Addictive patterns make us go into zombie mode, distracting us and keeping us from being present in the moment. Set the intention and ask for help from the Wise Witness to *be present* when an eating compulsion strikes. By setting this intention, you commit to your own healing and plant your feet squarely on Recovery Road. It's as if you're saying, "I'm ready to move on and transform my dysfunctional relationship with food." After you've set the intention to be present, even if you continue to go unconscious the next 20, 50, or 500 times the impulse to eat comes up, something in you will remember that intention, and eventually you'll be able to interrupt the emotional food-stuffing response. The more often you can interrupt your usual pattern, the easier it will become. Just as you created the old habit of eating in response to frightening and uncomfortable emotions, you can create a new habit of awareness by slowing down the action and removing yourself from the danger zone—wherever the food is.

80.

When a craving is on the scene, it can feel like it's driving and we're just along for the ride. When we finally fulfill our desire, finally bite into that donut or piece of chocolate cake, we *credit the food* for the momentary bliss we feel. But we have it backwards. *It's the craving that caused the suffering*, not our being deprived of the object of our desire. And *it's the elimination of the craving that caused the bliss,* not the food. We feel great because we're no longer burdened by the craving, yet we mistakenly give the credit to the chocolate cake. If we overeat the chocolate cake, the suffering isn't really gone, but transformed into the guilt and self-loathing we feel after indulging. The ego keeps our thinking compartmentalized so that in the throes of a craving, we think only about the object of our desire, not the complete experience. We become the Scarlett O'Haras of eating, opining, "I'll think about that tomorrow." This is how we dupe ourselves into indulging and suffering again and again. We think only about the fleeting pleasure we get from fulfilling the craving and ignore the negative repercussions.

81.

Here's the ego's version of following a craving versus the complete experience:

> **The Ego's Version:** *Craving → Obtaining the Object of Desire → Fulfillment*
>
> **The Complete Experience:** *Craving → Indulgence → Momentary Pleasure Due to Elimination of the Desire → Guilt, Self-Loathing, and Weight Gain.*

When a craving hits we fool ourselves when we tell ourselves that we can just have a little of what we desire and then stop. But if we're addicted to a food, it's very difficult to stick to that plan. Most of us end up overeating because we don't find the satisfaction we expect, and there's no clear signal to stop other than the pain of an overstuffed belly. Healing is about telling yourself the truth. If you could eat just a little of something you crave, you wouldn't suffer the physical, emotional, and spiritual consequences that often go hand in hand with addictive pleasures. You would break the cycle and take your power back. Unfortunately, most people with food issues can't do this.

82.

When you hear that familiar voice inside your head demanding "I want to eat this now," you can be sure the Child is on the scene. The wise adult part of us wants to eat a particular food because it's part of our nutritional agenda for the day. The Child gets us into trouble, and the more we can recognize her, the less power she has over us. Every time you decide not to respond to the child, you reduce its power. The more you can recognize the Child aspect of yourself, the easier it will be to align with the Wise Witness and take your power back. The Wise Witness knows there's a price to pay for following this pleasure-seeking principle, and if you strengthen your Wise Witness by listening to it more, you will feel less compelled to follow the dictates of the Child.

83.

When the desire to eat pleasure food arises, just recognize it: "Oh, that's the Child." Doing this lessens the Child's power because, all of a sudden, you realize that what you thought you wanted is really just what the Child wants. In seeing this, you've dis-identified with the Child. When you see the truth, it interrupts the pattern and cuts through it. The two benefits of dis-identifying with the Child are that it weakens the ego and leaves you with time to make a more rational choice. Instead of indulging, you might say, "I'm not going to indulge the Child right now." Or, like a wise parent, you might just say "no" to it: "No, you can't have another cookie." Or, from a place of choice and detachment, you might decide, "Okay, let's have some pleasure." In that case, you're choosing rather than reacting based on compulsion.

84.

When you react out of habit, it feels like you have no choice. But when you're aligned with the Wise Witness, you're free to make a choice. When you're listening to and obeying the Child, you're bound. That's a huge difference! The goal is to recognize that you're not the Child and develop enough distance from her so that you're free from unconsciously acquiescing to her and indulging her demands. When you see that the "I" that craves is the ego and *not you*, it is much easier to ignore a craving. You become *that which is noticing the Child craving food*. From that place of dis-identification, you can turn your attention elsewhere. Don't be discouraged if, in the beginning, noticing food thoughts is still followed by eating. The pattern of following your thoughts into the kitchen may be deeply entrenched. Fortunately, if you're patient and vigilant, noticing these food thoughts will eventually lead to being able to ignore them.

85.

Emotional eating is eating without being completely aware that you're eating. Instead, you're thinking and feeling—and feeding your feelings with—stressful thoughts while semi-consciously shoveling down copious quantities of food, perhaps without even tasting it. The strength of your eating compulsion is due to the countless times you've reinforced it by reaching for food to soothe uncomfortable emotions. But fear not! It's possible to interrupt this pattern, using powerful kung fu exercises. You just need to pick the one that you think will be the easiest for you to use. Pretty soon, using your kung fu will become automatic and that habit will replace your old habit of emotional eating.

86.

Powerful Kung Fu #1: Dis-identify with the Feeling. Ask yourself, "What am I feeling right now?" Wait for the answer. When the answer comes, ask yourself, "**What is noticing [the particular feeling you are feeling]?**" Fill in the blank with whatever feeling is present. Let's say agitation is present. Ask yourself, "What is noticing agitation?" This question helps you dis-identify with the feeling. Or say to yourself, "**It's just [the particular feeling]. What a relief. It's not me. It couldn't be me because I'm over here, noticing it.**" It's such a huge relief to realize that the feeling is not you! Normally we merge with negative feelings and assume they're *our* feelings, but they belong to the ego, not to us—not to who we really are. When we identify with the feeling, we have little power or objectivity. But when we notice a feeling, we're outside of it, aligned with the Wise Witness. In my experience, this kung fu cuts the power of the feeling in half immediately.

87.

Powerful Kung Fu #2: Allow the Feeling to Be There. Drop your story about the feeling and simply allow it to be there. Notice the sensation. What does it feel like in your body? Allow the feeling to be there without any agenda for it to dissipate. Accepting it and allowing it to be present will enable it to eventually dissolve. Emotions don't come to stay; they come to leave. If you can learn to stop feeding them with more negative thoughts, they dissolve more quickly. The best internal posture is simply to be present and allow whatever is happening in the moment, without adding more negative thoughts to it. Ask yourself, **"Can I just allow [the particular feeling] to be here?"**

88.

Powerful Kung Fu #3: Identify the Need. Ask yourself, **"What am I needing right now that is causing me to want some pleasure?"** If the answer is appreciation, comfort, or understanding, in your imagination, give yourself what you need—a hug or words of consolation or praise. Alternatively, ask yourself, **"Is there something else here that's whole and complete and doesn't need anything?"** This will help you see the real you, the you that doesn't actually need what you may think you need.

89.

Powerful Kung Fu #4: Is There Something I Need to Address? Ask yourself, **"Is there something I need to address inside myself, with another person, or in my life?"** Get curious about what that could be and be prepared for insights to arise. Then, take action to address any disharmonies or imbalances.

90.

Powerful Kung Fu #5: Dis-identify with the Troublesome Food Thought. Ask yourself, "What is it that is aware of the thought 'I want food right now'?" Next, ask, "Is that thought or impulse to eat really me? If I am aware of it, how can it be me?" Once you realize that this thought is not you, you automatically dis-identify with it, and it loses its power.

91.

Powerful Kung Fu #6: The Mosquito Flick. Notice that an impractical food thought is on the scene and imagine flicking it away, the same way you would flick away an annoying mosquito.

92.

Powerful Kung Fu #7: Notice that the Child Is on the Scene.Tell yourself, "Oh, that's just the Child. No big deal. For a minute there, I thought I wanted to eat something, but it was just what the Child wanted. She wanted to distract me. Thank goodness it's just the Child and not me."

93.

Powerful Kung Fu #8: See the Whole Picture of Food. Remember the whole picture of food. The pleasure of eating a particular food is so short-lived! Imagine how bad you will feel if you overeat.

94.

Powerful Kung Fu #9: Put Your Attention on Something Else. Do or think about something else. Read a book. Talk to someone. Take a walk. Do a crossword puzzle. Finish the laundry. Drive somewhere. Turn on the television. Listen to music. Meditate. Focus on your senses. What are you feeling, seeing, smelling, or hearing? Almost any distraction will do. Make a list of noneating activities you find engaging and nurturing so that when a craving strikes, you're ready for it.Don't give your attention to ego-based thoughts (especially negative ones), thoughts that are about "me" or "my story" or that start with "I," such as "I like, I want, I don't want, I hope, I don't like, I feel, I think, I believe, I can't, I won't, I'm not, I did..." This involvement with the "me" is what gave you the craving crazies in the first place.

95.

Powerful Kung Fu #10: Get Engaged in What You're Doing. Become engaged and focus completely on whatever you're doing now, whether it's work, running an errand, vacuuming, finishing a good book, or making a call. When you're really absorbed in something, you can go for hours without a single thought about food.

96.

Powerful Kung Fu #11: Pick a "9" or "10" Think of something that you love to do, a "9" or "10." Take a break from whatever was causing your hand to reach for food and do something you love instead.

97.

Powerful Kung Fu #12: I Do that, Too. If you're angry or feel hurt because someone did something you didn't like, remember a time that you did or said the same sort of thing and forgive that person. It's hard to stay angry at someone when we find the same failing in ourselves. To keep yourself from stuffing the feeling with food and heal instead, see your own failing, and forgive yourself and the other person.

98.

Powerful Kung Fu #13: Dis-identify with the Stressful Thought. Ask yourself, **"What stressful thought am I believing right now?"** or **"What story am I in?"** Wait for the answer.When the answer comes, ask yourself, **"What is noticing this belief?"** This is a powerful question because it helps you dis-identify with the thought.Say to yourself, **"Oh, thank goodness, it's just a stressful belief—it's not me. It couldn't be me because I'm over here, noticing it."**

99.

Powerful Kung Fu #14: Inquire. Notice that you're upset and address the upset directly using inquiry. Do this by asking yourself, **"What story am I telling myself that's causing me to feel this way right now? What am I believing?"**When you discover the belief, take it to inquiry by asking the following questions:**Can I know beyond a shadow of a doubt that this belief is true?** Even if you believe that it's true, go on to the next question.**What is the opposite of this belief? Could that be as true or truer?** Come up with evidence to support the opposite belief. If the opposite of the belief is also true, perhaps the original negative belief isn't true after all! This discovery helps you to stop believing the stressful thought.

100.

Powerful Kung Fu #15: Think Something Positive Instead. Replace the negative thought that's generating the feeling with a positive one. For example, replace "Nothing's going right today." with "Everything's going right today." Then come up with evidence to support the positive thought. This kung fu can be a bit of a slippery slope because it does keep you in the realm of thought, and when you're in thought, it's easy to go back to spinning a negative story and feeding the feeling again.

101.

Powerful Kung Fu #16: Not Now—Maybe Later. Recognize that the Child is on the scene and talk to her the way you would talk to a child who is pestering you about getting something that you don't want to give her right now. Tell her, **"Not now—maybe later."**

102.

Powerful Kung Fu #17: Just This Once…Rather than treading the well-worn path of self-soothing through food, try something different just this once. Don't give in to the usual urge—for now. You can always decide to do that later, if that's what you want, but for now, move out of the kitchen.

103.

Powerful Kung Fu #18: Am I Hungry? (The Cottage Cheese Test) Ask yourself if you are physically hungry. This is different than just wanting to taste something nice. One of my workshop participants uses what she calls "the cottage cheese test." She likes cottage cheese, but the only time she actually wants to eat it is when she's truly hungry. If she could eat cottage cheese, she knows she's hungry. If she couldn't eat cottage cheese and she wants to eat something, she knows that she's not physically hungry and something else is going on. If you answer no when you ask yourself if you're physically hungry, ask yourself, **"What's going on that's causing me to want to move toward food when I'm not hungry?"**

Pick the kung fu for cravings and emotional eating works that works best for you and do a dress rehearsal. Imagine having a craving and using the your trusty kung fu to knock it out.

104.

Here's the whole truth of overeating pleasure food: It comes out to 5% "taste good" (for the few short minutes that it spends in your mouth) and 95% bloat, weight gain, ill health, guilt, shame, blame, self-deprecation, and perpetual low self-esteem. Once you really saw this, you can no longer pretend that you hadn't seen it. Once you stop believing in Santa Claus, you can't just decide to believe in him again. The jig is up. It may take many repetitions of seeing the whole truth of overeating in the midst of a compulsive impulse finally be able to interrupt it. Please be gentle and patient with yourself!

105.

Remember to see the whole truth about food rather than the Child's sliver of truth about it. Remember all of the unpleasant consequences of overeating a pleasure food:

Feeling guilty about eating unhealthily and not being strong enough to stop,

Ill health

Not fitting into clothes

Wanting to hide because you feel too fat

Weight gain

Low self-esteem

Losing confidence professionally and socially

Feeling bloated, nauseated, or listless.

106.

If you're willing to see that an irrational part of yourself has been running the show, then you can begin to develop a more rational approach to eating. Today, focus on distinguishing between the problematic thoughts that come from the Child and the pragmatic thoughts that come from the Wise Witness. See if you can successfully ignored a thought from the Child.

107.

Today spend some time feeding your soul. And make a plan to spend some time feeding your soul each day this week. Remember to be gentle and patient with yourself when if you indulge a craving or engaged in emotional eating. If you aren't able to be tender with yourself over the next few days, notice that tendency to be harsh, set the intention to be kinder to yourself next time, and forgave yourself.

108.

What are some of your "9's" and "10's," the things you love to do. Make sure to spend even a few minutes today and every day doing a "9" or a "10."

109.

Making wise food choices means getting most of your calories from healthy, nutritious, whole foods like fruit, vegetables, seeds, nuts, grains, and meats—eventually. What is your "eventually?" What is your timetable for change? The sooner you start implementing the Second Step, the easier and happier your life will be. Making wise food choices also means eating with health in mind—eating foods that make sense for the optimal functioning of your body. It's common sense. Every day, you'll want to make sure you get protein, carbohydrates, and healthy fats from whole, unprocessed foods. Ideally, each meal would be balanced in this way, too. The body is adaptable, and it's okay to eat for pleasure sometimes as long as *eventually* most of your calories are nutritious calories. If you're not sure how to eat healthily, read a good book on nutrition.

110.

When you're hungry, rather than imagining what would taste good right now, go to your rational mind and ask, "What could my body use right now?" If you haven't been eating or thinking about food this way, it's not surprising. Our culture doesn't support this way of thinking about food. It tends to encourage the Child's romanticization of food.

111.

We know deep down that our bodies run on whole food, but we continue to feed them junk. We seek the taste pleasure of nonfoods like candy, cookies, donuts, and potato chips and at the same time we want to strut around in sexy, thin bodies. The problem is that bodies that eat junk get fat, sluggish, moody, and sick, just as cars that are filled with the wrong fuel don't run well or seize up. It's a simple law of mechanics.

112.

Food is grown or raised and contains nutrients that the body needs. *Junk is made*. It's processed and refined, designed primarily to tantalize our palates. This is an important distinction to keep in mind.

113.

Marketers have been co-opted by the ego, which makes them the mouthpiece of the Child. Her main job when it comes to food is getting us to eat entertaining food, enticing us based on the imagined taste pleasure food delivers. With pleasure food, you experience the intense pleasure hit while the food is in your mouth, but then what? To keep that sensation going, you need to take another bite and then another, and so on. At some point, those bites don't taste very good, and your stomach protests. The pleasure turns into pain. The attraction turns into repulsion. As your body struggles to digest the junk, you feel bloated, headachy, groggy, and grumpy. Your body suffers because not only did it not receive the nutrients it needs, it now has to expend precious energy to get rid of the junk. To top it off, it may have to carry around excess weight as a result of this pleasure food party.

114.

The bottom line is this: If you want to avoid the pull of the Child and negate her influence on your eating life, avoid sexy food ads. Turn away from any images or sound bites that quicken your pulse and get you salivating. When the Child encourages you to imagine what food tastes like, ignore those thoughts. If you follow them, you may find yourself careening down a slippery slope and landing smack-dab in the middle of an over-the-top pleasure food party.

115.

Generally, the pleasure foods that you can't stop eating have—surprise, surprise—almost no nutrition. You couldn't survive on them. As a culture, we've fooled ourselves into thinking that pleasure food is food, but it's not. It's entertainment. Don't delude yourself into thinking that the junk you're ingesting is food. If you do, you're going to replace real food with entertaining junk and think you're getting the nutrition you need. You might be getting a tiny bit of nutrition from it, but even that comes at a very high cost.

116.

If you see pleasure food as entertainment, you'll be less likely to replace good food with it, and it will hold a smaller place in your life. Just like you don't watch television all day long or go to the movies every night because you have other things to do, it's unhealthy to eat pleasure food too often. You watch a television show at night or go to a movie once a week. Similarly, maybe you have a little pleasure food at night or make a conscious decision to entertain yourself with it one night a week.

117.

Eating Processed Fast Food Means Choosing Taste over Health. Most restaurants use considerably more fat, salt, and sugar than we would at home. A restaurant's motive is profit, not our health, and creating food that tastes better than the competition's is the key to filling its coffers. If we're to bring our bodies back into balance, though, we need to ask ourselves, "Is taste more important than health?"

118.

We've been focused on taste from the time we were children, and our taste buds have become accustomed to the flavors of pleasure foods, expecting them every time we eat. But now that we're adults, it's time to take responsibility for our eating and tell ourselves the truth: Most food companies and restaurants sell unhealthy foods that human bodies were never designed to eat, and if we want to get healthy and stay at a natural weight, we have to stop or limit our junk eating.

119.

If you're overweight, you're probably eating a lot of fat and sugar, perhaps more than you even know, which dramatically throws off your metabolism and your relationship to food. It's difficult to comprehend the full impact of this way of eating because you're accustomed to it and, to a certain extent, your body has adapted to it. To reverse this unnatural trend, you've got to eliminate most of the junk in favor of fresh, whole, unprocessed foods. *You don't need to become rigid or completely pure in your eating.* The body is adaptable and can handle most foods if you don't inundate it with processed stuff. Giving it the appropriate amount of produce and whole, natural foods reacclimates your taste buds to the food you were designed to eat. Once that happens, eating healthily becomes easy and—believe it or not—preferable! Why? Because you end up enjoying nutritious foods more than you ever enjoyed the junk. Also, when you reduce the amount of fat, salt, and sugar you're consuming, the difference in your energy level and feeling of well-being is dramatic.

120.

Not only do food companies make food that we can't stop eating, *they have remade us.* Eating their addictive products rewired our taste buds and metabolisms. The companies created the products and now those same products have re-created us to be their perfect consumers. Food, which was once nice-tasting fuel for the body, has become a much bigger deal. It has become a celebrity, a superstar, a guilty pleasure of biblical proportions. The questions you have to ask yourself are: Do I want food to loom so large in my life? Do I want it to dominate my waking consciousness? Is there more to life than lusting after, craving, and avoiding food? If somewhere deep down in the recesses of your consciousness, you know that living this way is not really living, but indentured servitude, it's time to get your power back.

121.

Once you start getting most of your calories from healthy food, food that's grown, not made, you will find that it tastes every bit as good as pleasure food used to. In other words, you haven't given up anything!

122.

Ask yourself, "How important is freedom to me? Is it more important than a fleeting good taste in my mouth?" What is it like when you eat something that tastes nice for a few seconds but makes you feel out of control? Is it worth it?

123.

A skinny junk-food eater might not gain weight, but her body pays for this practice with diminished energy levels or a compromised immune system. The double whammy is a dangerous strategy for balancing the two mutually exclusive egoic desires of wanting to look good and wanting to eat our favorite pleasure foods. Even skinny junk-food eaters can only fool the body for so long. Sooner or later, everybody pays the price.

124.

Remember the whole truth when you are faced with eating a lot of pleasure food when you aren't hungry—it feels better to feel better longer. The Child plays the same game with us over and over again until we get wise to it. She hooks us with a small sliver of truth—pleasure food tastes good—and leaves out the rest of the truth. There is a place for eating entertaining food. But if we want to maintain healthy, slim bodies without worry or struggle, then that place is a small place. To feel better longer, we need to get the bulk of our calories from healthy, whole foods like fruits, vegetables, and whole grains, not from pleasure foods.

125.

Why Wait for Health Issues? Health scares can be so traumatic that we do an about-face in our eating. Oddly enough, when this happens, good fortune is smiling on us. Nothing helps us prioritize health faster than the prospect of the grim reaper knocking at our door. But do we really need to wait for a crisis? Why not embrace the possibility of choosing health over taste now? Doesn't waking up to the truth of how we're feeding our bodies *before* a health scare strikes make sense?

126.

Listening to our bodies to decide how to eat doesn't work these days because we're eating the wrong foods. The messages from a body that's addicted to junk are simply not a reliable guide to healthy eating. Pleasure food was created to entice us to eat it and throw off our taste buds and our body's signals for hunger and satiation. The truth is, as nice as the idea sounds, we really can't talk to our bodies. Although our bodies have some unconscious input into our eating—like when my girlfriend was anemic during her pregnancy and dreamt of liver sausage—we can't pick up the phone and dial our bodies to ask for guidance about what to eat. We can't communicate with our bodies on a conscious level.

127.

When you have an emotional relationship with a food, you crave it and feel giddy and excited around it. You may feel a frenzied compulsion to eat it not five minutes from now, but right now! Stressful thoughts about your relationship to this food undermine your self-esteem and cause even more destruction by triggering your conditioned pattern of eating it when you're upset.

128.

Although you probably already have a good idea about which foods make you feel out of control, it's helpful to clearly identify them. Use the following questions to see if you're on the right track. Start by filling in the blanks with "celery": Does the prospect of eating _____ make you giddy and excited? Do you have a hard time limiting how much _____ you eat? Can you easily eat just one bite and stop? Does eating _____ or having it around make you feel powerless and out of control? People generally don't get addicted to celery, carrots, or Brussels sprouts; they get addicted to junk.

129.

Seeing your relationship with food as a conditioned one that you formed as a child can help you begin to develop the more rational, adult part of you. You can say to yourself, "Oh yes, I can see that I've been conditioned to see that as a reward, but you know what? I've had enough rewards today, and I don't need to keep going in that direction. That's not good for my body." Conditioning creates an overblown relationship with food, causing us to see it as our lover, our friend, and our source of fulfillment. As a result, we think we need it to be happy. But we don't. Once you begin to see that, you can choose to change your relationship by questioning your beliefs. Acknowledging that your conditioning is causing you to sacrifice your health and emotional well-being means you can no longer be fooled by it. You step outside of it and move beyond your conditioning rather than continuing to react to it. From that place, there is freedom. There is choice.

130.

Thinking of food as a reward is only a problem if you reward yourself too much. When there's no parent there to say, "Hey, honey, you've had enough cookies," the Child says, "Whoopee! There's nobody here to stop me, so I can have as many cookies as I want." But every Child needs a parent. Just because you're grown up and there isn't an adult telling you when to stop doesn't mean you can eat whatever you want and not pay a price. If you want to permanently solve your weight and food issues, you need to develop the adult inside of you, or that Child's just going to keep chasing after the treats.

131.

Most of us experience having a more mature relationship with food when we're on a diet. At those times, the diet book becomes the parent. But unless you integrate that parent, you'll go back to your old ways as soon as the diet's over. You have to build a relationship with your own inner parent, your Wise Witness. Your Wise Witness is an aspect of yourself that has always been there, but you may not have noticed it because you were so busy listening to the Child. It's that objective place within you that is able to choose to follow your conditioning or not. The more often you align with the Wise Witness, the easier it becomes. The spiritual aspect of healing your food issues includes developing the sense of yourself as this Wise Witness who sees the whole picture, isn't buffeted by conditioning, and can choose whether to indulge or not.

132.

Why would we do something as irrational as eating food that has no nutritional value? Because it tastes good. We crave the taste, and how do we stop wanting what we want? The simple answer is that we can't. We can't push against desire because we're always too late. The only way to stop *wanting* a food is to decide that it's no longer in your life. Then you stop thinking about it and, if you're not thinking about it, you can't desire it. Here's how this works: Imagine that you're walking by a bakery with a friend. She wants a cookie and asks if you want one, too. You respond, "You go ahead. I don't eat cookies anymore." For most of us, a namby-pamby stance like "I'll cut down first," or "I'll give it up for Lent," just won't work. If you know you're going back to it, you'll be thinking about it, lighting candles for it, and holding all-night vigils awaiting its return.

133.

We like to tell ourselves that we can eat pleasure food in moderation. We're not wimps, after all. Just look at all the successful diets we've been on! We're grown-ups, and we can control ourselves around these foods that have become the main way we treat ourselves and get pleasure in life. And that's true—except when it isn't, when we lose it and overeat in response to a physical or emotional craving. We need to get real about this if we want a sane relationship with food. If we are ever to overcome our addiction, we need to face the music and take back our power over food. If you feel out of control over a certain food, either limit it using a strategy that works for you, or cut it out of your life.

134.

The more you eat any pleasure food, the more you want it, and the more you want it, the more you eat it. It's a vicious circle. Although it seems counterintuitive, the only way to stop wanting a food is to stop eating it. Here's why: When you stop eating the food and decide that it's out of your life forever—not just for a day or a week or a month—you stop thinking about it. When you stop thinking about it, you stop desiring it. We're used to thinking, "Gosh, if I stop eating this food that I love, I'll feel deprived and want it all the more." This is true if you cut out pleasure foods temporarily, but *if you decide that certain foods are no longer in your life, you stop thinking about them.* And if you stop thinking about them, you stop craving them. If you stop craving them, you stop eating them, and—wonder of wonders—you lose weight! It takes thought to create desire. No thought, no desire. It's just that simple.

135.

Giving up pleasure foods demands a colossal massing of willpower. Thank goodness that's not true. If it were, I'd be in big trouble! The good news is that it's actually *easier* to give up the junk than to keep eating it. When we decide not to let a particular food past our lips ever again, we effectively shut the door on the egoic mind, the source of impractical food thoughts. Hence, to stop cravings, we need to turn away from thoughts about the foods we crave. When we keep eating nonfood, we make it so hard on ourselves! But if we decide that a food like chocolate is no longer in our lives, we may miss it for a day or two, but then we forget about it—no pain, no feeling of deprivation. On the other hand, when we go on a diet and expect to be able to eat our coveted foods again on the maintenance plan, we end up counting down the days until maintenance time arrives. If thoughts arise about a food that you've given up, simply ignore them. Don't, I repeat, *don't* give them an audience. If you spend a lot of time entertaining your thoughts about that food, you'll torture yourself. Give up the food for good, commit to not spending any time thinking about it, and life will be so much more pleasant.

136.

Given all the trouble that pleasure foods create in terms of disease and overweight, it's clear that our bodies weren't designed to eat them. If you think of it that way, it's easier to eliminate certain foods. If you're still resisting this change, though, because it's hard for you to imagine yourself eating primarily nutritious foods, it's totally natural. Don't worry about it. However, what you can't really know until you've put abstinence into practice is that *you're not really giving up anything.* You're just establishing a different relationship to food, one that's more wholesome, freer, and less obsessive. The reason abstaining from pleasure food works is because you don't eliminate the pleasure of eating; you simply *eliminate eating food solely for pleasure.* That's a big difference. Even if you eliminate all of your favorite foods (and I'm by no means suggesting you do that), you'll still get pleasure from eating because food tastes good, and even healthy food is pleasurable to eat.

137.

The bulk of current diet wisdom tells us not to ever let ourselves feel deprived because if we limit ourselves, we'll overeat later. The truth is that you can't continue to eat whatever you want, particularly the addictive foods, if you want to be free from your challenging relationship with food. You've done that, and you know it doesn't work. By not depriving yourself of these foods, you're trying to appease the Child so that she doesn't cajole you into eating everything that's not nailed down. But when you align with the Wise Witness, you recognize that the Child is using the idea of deprivation as a ploy, and you learn to stop listening to her. In this way, you break free from your conditioning rather than trying to manage it.

138.

Try asking yourself, "What is it that will feel deprived if I give up an addictive food—my body or me? Is it true that my body will feel deprived? Or is it truer that I'm fantasizing about having a certain taste experience?" The truth is that the body won't feel deprived, the ego will. The Child will. Deprivation is a conditioned idea that the Child has talked to us about so many times that we've actually come to believe it.

139.

The Child tells us that we're feeling deprived, so we deserve two slices of chocolate mousse cake and a hot fudge sundae. She uses the idea of deprivation as an excuse for overeating, and we comply. The body, on the other hand, couldn't care less. It eats whatever is in front of it. Deprivation is a conditioned idea that tells us we should be able to expect certain taste experiences because we've had them in the past. If we're used to having dessert, we come to expect it, and when we don't have it, we tell ourselves the story of "being deprived" and get in a tizzy about it. Deprivation is a lie that the Child tells you. It's how we characterize the Child's tantrum when her desire for pleasure food is not being met. Once you see this, you're on to the ego's game, and you can't be tricked into believing in or following the lie. You're no longer attached to getting pleasure from pleasure food. When you're free from that attachment, you still enjoy food as much, if not more than, before, but *you no longer need to get pleasure from a particular food at a particular time.*

140.

In transitioning to healthier foods, it's helpful to identify a few foods that you don't have an addictive relationship with that you consider treats. Find foods that you don't want to keep eating and eating once you start. If, at any point, you discover that you can't stop eating them, eliminate them— that is, if you want to be free of the addictive relationship. How do you know whether you can have just a little bit of a treat food? If you can set a rule for yourself about it and stick to it, then it's a treat food you can moderate. You can't leave out the food component and expect to lick this issue. Sure, it would be nice to think that we could take off the weight and then eat whatever we wanted. But that's a pipe dream.

141.

The food industry isn't fighting fair. They design foods that are irresistible and, as much as we would like to, we can't moderate these foods. If we could moderate, we would have. We have to stop engaging in the kind of thinking that keeps us on the dieting, gaining, dieting treadmill. The costs to our self-esteem and our health are huge! Aren't you ready to stop this way of living?

142.

We think that choice is freedom, but the opposite is actually true. For people who are overly involved with food, *choice is bondage*. When I make an eating plan for myself, it may be true that I've eliminated spontaneity. But I've also eliminated the gut-wrenching internal debates over "Should I or shouldn't I indulge?" and blocked the Child's access point. If my decision is already made, she doesn't have a chance to sneak in and steer me toward the wrong foods and eating too much.

143.

Being able to eat whatever we want and as much as we want is a common fantasy. It's brought to us by none other than our good friend the Child and, surprise, surprise, it leads us in the direction of suffering. Imagining that other people get to eat whatever they want and not gain weight, we get jealous and decide we've been dealt a lousy hand in the card game of life.

144.

Imagine that you can eat as much junk as you want and stay thin. Here's what would happen: By playing out this fantasy, you're eating mostly junk, and there is no off switch for that stuff. The defining characteristics of junk are that it's not satisfying and you can't stop eating it. As a result, you're overfilling your stomach and feeling bloated, lethargic, and uncomfortable most days. Junk has little or no nutritional value. You're not giving your body the nutrition it needs, so you are becoming increasingly unhealthy. If sugar is in the mix, you're experiencing mood swings, and the people around you aren't about to award you any popularity prizes. Finally—and this is a big one—you feel out of control around junk. Of course, you may counter, "So what if I feel out of control? I can eat as much as I want, remember? That's the whole point of this fantasy." But feeling out of control around food is no fun. There's no freedom in it. It doesn't feel good to be addicted to a substance and not be able to stop consuming it. Being able to eat as much junk as we want is the booby prize!

145.

Weight loss is a tortoise and the hare race. There are no brownie points for being quick off the starting mark. Instead, it's about going the distance and getting a body that you'll like for life, not just for a few weeks. Your reward for deciding to eat healthy food most of the time is twofold: 1) a healthy body that stays at a natural weight, and 2) freedom—you won't have to struggle and suffer over feeling out of control around food.

146.

Eliminate foods you haven't been able to moderate or, at the very least, to not let them into your house. Know that when you eliminate something, it's out of your life for good. You can't be wishy-washy about it or it won't work. Once you cut one thing out, you'll see that it's not difficult to do. When you eliminate something, you stop thinking about it, which means you stop desiring it, and you don't suffer. Desire equals suffering. When you don't completely eliminate a food from your diet, you don't banish it from your thinking. And thinking about food is where all the trouble starts.

147.

Wise eating is learning to eat from a place of presence, balance, and calm rather than from a frenzied, out-of-control, mechanical, or can't-get-enough-of-this-heavenly-substance-called-food place. Many of us go "zombie" when we're eating and become oblivious to how much food is going in. Without knowing it, we shovel in food like we're the Energizer Bunny set loose in a carrot patch. Anything we can do to become aware of and interrupt this pattern is helpful.

148.

If you tend to race through meals, it's easy to overfill your stomach. It's amazing how many calories can go in when you're eating fast! Make a conscious effort to eat in slow motion and chew your food thoroughly. This is especially important when you're very hungry. Otherwise, the Child can get the upper hand and say, "I'm hungry. It's time to let loose and eat a lot!" When you're shoveling rather than eating, you can't enjoy your food nearly as much.

149.

Make eating a sitting-down activity. Eat with your tush in a chair and your food on a plate. Why? If you study your emotional eating habits, my hunch is that you'll discover that emotional eating often happens when you're standing up.

150.

Emotional eating happens in a hurry. We eat out of the fridge or pantry or over the sink or in the car when we're possessed by the "emotional-eating crazies." If you take the time to sit down and put your food on a plate, though, it helps you wake up and be more conscious of what you're doing. You can eat a lot of food when you're not paying attention. The Child tricks you into believing that if you're not paying attention, what you're eating doesn't count. So you believe that calories that come from nibbling don't count. But they do.

151.

Nibbling robs us of eating pleasure if we're eating while doing other things at the same time. Because my attention was divided, I couldn't completely enjoy the food or focus on my phone conversation or my cooking. And that was ultimately unsatisfying. To finally overcome this habit, I decided not to nibble for one day, just to see if I could do it. Then one day turned into two days, and so on. Why not give this a try? See if you can go one full day without nibbling.

152.

If food has been your drug of choice, you've used to it to numb out. That's been your habit. To get free, you need to create a new habit of being present during the experience of eating—to *just eat when you're eating*. See if you can stay awake while you eat. I'm not talking about not nodding off and falling into your soup. I'm talking about staying present and experiencing the sensations of eating rather than escaping into thought. For the ego, the problem with being fully present when we're eating is that it brings us into the moment. The sensation of eating, like any other sense experience, is a portal to your true self. Biting into an apple involves all five senses. If you bring your awareness to the sensations of eating, you can't help but be in the moment, aligned with your true self instead of the ego. And if you're out of the ego, you don't need it, and it's out of a job.

153.

To maintain a healthy weight, we need to educate ourselves about portion size. The truth is that *the portions we imagine we can eat are much larger than what we can actually eat without gaining weight*. It comes as no surprise that eating large portions means gaining weight. Find out what portion sizes are appropriate for you rather than accepting the heaping platefuls restaurants dole out.

154.

Do you know about how many calories you need to maintain a healthy weight? If you don't, consider working with a nutritionist to find out. Once you have an idea, translate that number into food choices and portion sizes. You can pick up a pocket calorie counter at your local bookstore or supermarket to help you with this. For example, find out what the portions look like in a 400- to 500-calorie meal and use that as a guide to help you eat more reasonable amounts. If you go to a restaurant, look at the portion you receive. Is it reasonable? If not, don't eat it all. Only eat the amount of food that you decide is appropriate.

155.

Assuming we can rely on our stomach to tell us how much food to eat is one of our main misconceptions. Judging from the feeling in our stomach after we've eaten a reasonable portion, we often think we're still hungry, so we eat more. But the feeling of satiation doesn't register right away after we've eaten, and for some people, it never registers.

156.

There are different degrees of hunger. If you're tummy-rumbling hungry, that's a trustworthy sign that it's time to eat a meal. But when you've already eaten, using *the feeling in your stomach* to tell you how much more to eat or when to stop *is an unreliable gauge*. Sometimes the more we eat, the hungrier we feel! If the body were good at telling people when to stop eating, there wouldn't be so many obese people around. Although the sensations in your stomach might be a gross measure of whether you're hungry enough to eat a meal, they don't tell you when to put on the brakes. *Let portion size, rather than the feeling in your stomach, determine how much you eat.*

157.

To maintain a natural, healthy weight, we need to learn to tolerate some hunger before we eat a meal. Hunger is a good friend who's been given a bad rap. If you let it, it can help you end your weight battle for good. See whether it's possible to welcome some hunger and allow it to be there for a short time rather than sprinting to the fridge the minute you notice you're no longer full. Maintaining a normal body size means learning to live with some hunger, and not being willing to embrace hunger means living in a heavier body. If you're not comfortable with this idea, look at your beliefs about it. Perhaps you're giving hunger more meaning than it warrants. Does it stir up fears that you're not going to survive? Begin by abandoning the notion that *you know* about hunger. Get curious about the experience. Welcome it and see what it actually is, as opposed to what you think it is. To help your unconscious ideas surface, ask yourself why hunger is so frightening or uncomfortable. What are your beliefs about it? What will happen if you let yourself get hungry? On a separate sheet of paper or in your journal, list your fears and beliefs. What are the meanings you've given hunger? What stories do you tell yourself that cause you to reach frantically for anything edible to immediately quell any hunger sensations?

158.

Today, each time you feel a hunger sensation, ask yourself, "Am I hungry?" When you're hungry, wait 30 minutes or an hour before eating. When you do this, you may notice that the hunger comes and goes, and the most uncomfortable feelings don't last. If you ignore them and don't fill them with food right away, they turn into other sensations that are easier to live with. At some point, hunger sensations level off or even disappear rather than getting worse and worse. After your day of experimenting with hunger, compare your experiences with the fears and beliefs you listed earlier. Were your negative assumptions about hunger true?

159.

I'll let you in on a little secret: The ego is always seeking comfort. The prospect of discomfort, no matter how small, sends it scurrying for the exit. Hunger is no exception. The ego says, "Why should I experience the discomfort of hunger if I don't have to? Life throws me enough curveballs already, but hunger isn't one of them. I don't *have* to feel hunger, so I'm not gonna!" Have you ever considered that hunger might be an aspect of the divine plan, integral to the optimal functioning of the body? Like eating, resting, and exercising, perhaps bodies need to experience hunger to run well. Could it be that hunger is how the body supports us in maintaining a healthy size?

160.

Have you noticed how delicious food tastes when you're hungry? Even a carrot tastes like manna from heaven. When you allow yourself to get tummy-rumbling hungry, you enjoy your food in a way that isn't possible when your tank is full. When you're not full, but not quite hungry either, the taste of food and the experience of eating are not nearly as satisfying. Think of your body like a car. You don't indiscriminately pull your car up to the gas pump. When you see the fuel gauge getting close to empty, you start looking for a gas station. In the same way, check if your stomach tank is genuinely empty before you fill it. Ask yourself if you're really hungry. If not, wait until you feel the growling in your stomach that means the body needs food. This sounds simple, yet most of us rarely wait for that signal. If you're serious about having a more balanced and sane relationship with food, begin to live with some hunger and wait to eat until you feel it.

161.

Although the general rule of thumb is to eat only when you're hungry, there is a qualification: Eat only when you're hungry, and *only if it's also when you've decided that you will eat*. If you've been overeating on a regular basis, it's important initially that you not follow the dictates of your stomach because overeating has thrown off your appetite, and it needs to readjust before you can trust your hunger. Your stomach sensations are unbalanced in proportion to how unbalanced your relationship is to food. You may think, "But I'm so hungry," but you've trained your body to be hungry frequently by feeding it often. In this case, it's helpful to come up with an eating plan that provides a reasonable number of calories, spread throughout the day, and use it as your guide.

162.

One of the easiest ways to release negative ideas is to replace them with positive ones. Here are some positive thoughts to help you counter the ego's negative commentary:

Hunger is good.

Hunger is normal.

Hunger is helping me reset my taste buds and my metabolism.

Hunger is easy to tolerate.

Hunger is healthy.

Hunger is welcome here.

Hunger is freeing me.

Hunger is helping me to reach a healthy weight.

Wow! I experienced hunger and I lived!

My body is designed to get hungry before it eats.

163.

In the ego's world, there is always duality—pleasure seeking carries within it the seed of pain. The ego doesn't tell us that, of course, because we would be less likely to follow a promise of pleasure that also leads to pain. So it tries to hook us with the pleasant half of the story and avoids the unpleasant half. If you want to maintain a natural, healthy weight, you can't keep your old habits. You can't continue to eat the same foods you've been eating and not monitor portion size. Let me repeat so this is crystal clear: You can't ever go back to eating what you've been eating. You can't ever go back to not monitoring portion size. You can't ever go back to eating when you're not hungry. Thinking you can return to your old habits is the kind of deluded, egoic thinking that has kept you yo-yoing over the years. Following your true self's impulses toward health and balance have no cost, no downside. In creating new, healthy habits, you don't give up anything. The pleasure is there as much as ever, if not more so, because there's no inner conflict. Not only will you reach a healthy weight, you'll get to keep your new body without struggle or worry for the rest of your life. It's a win-win.

164.

If food has been your primary source of pleasure, parties can be a huge challenge. How do you keep the wise, rational part of you in charge? What's in the Wise Witness's arsenal to fortify you in the face of these powerful temptations? Two words—a plan. A plan can be as simple as "I will limit myself to healthy food and reasonable portions." It can be something you pen the day before or commit to five minutes before you leave for the party. Plans put the wise part of you in charge and keep the Child at bay. The Child will fight you on this because she doesn't like to commit. She'll say things like, "What if I want a few cheese puffs? What's wrong with that? Why do I have to plan that? Can't I just eat like a normal person?! Is this how life is going to be? I'm going to have to *plan* everything from now until I die?!" Ignore her. Here are two suggestions for making a party plan.

Decide ahead of time that this party is not an eating event for you.

Decide ahead of time to eat at the party, but to eat only the foods and portions that you designate. Put your food on a single plate and limit your party eating to only what is on that plate—that food and nothing more.

Contrary to the advice in many books on eating and weight issues, it's okay to take your bathroom scale out of storage. The ego doesn't want us to weigh ourselves because it doesn't want to know the truth. This is not only how it deals with food and weight—but with all of life! It wants to pretend it can do whatever it wants without accountability, and the scale represents nothing if not accountability.

165.

Imagining how food tastes is a slippery slope that leaves you vulnerable to backsliding (going off the plan you've made for yourself). When you imagine how something will taste, you create a desire for it. It's dangerous. Once a desire is generated, it begs to be fulfilled. Planning eliminates imagining. When you plan what to eat for the day, you eliminate the option of imagining and fantasizing about other foods, so desires for those foods aren't created. You also eliminate desire for what you are going to eat. If you know what you're going to eat, there's nothing to desire. You can't desire what you already have because *desire comes from wanting what you don't have.* The ego resists committing to a plan with all its might. It's wishy-washy. "*Maybe* I'll do this," it says, or, "*I'll try* to do that." The problem with this approach is that it, too, leaves you vulnerable to backsliding because you didn't *really* commit. Whenever you notice you're unwilling to commit to a plan you've created, that's the ego trying to sabotage your intentions to eat well.

166.

"What if I'm in situations where I can't plan, and I'm forced to accept the food that's available?" Simple. As soon as you know what's available, create a plan within those parameters. You can say to yourself, "Okay, here's what's available. I don't have to put every food I see on my plate just because it's here. I can pick and choose what and how much to eat." If you just start eating without thinking about what you're doing or creating a plan, you start to slide down the slippery slope. Here's how the Wise Witness deals with going out to eat: "We're going to a restaurant, and they serve buffet style, so I'll have a fist-sized portion of protein and fill the rest of my plate with vegetables. I'll eat that, and only that, and not return for seconds." Here's how the Wise Witness might plan for a trip: "I'm traveling, and I need to bring enough food to last the 18-hour journey, so I'll eat X at this time and Y at that time." Or, "I'll be driving all day in an area that only offers fast food, so I'll bring healthy food with me. That way, I won't have to eat food that's not good for me." You know that you can commit, plan, and strategize because you've done it many times when you've dieted. You simply ignore the Child, who always wants to thwart your plans. When most of us go off a diet, however, we let the Child start guiding our eating again. That's why we regain the weight we lost.

167.

The Child hates eating pragmatically; she always wants to be free to do what she wants, when she wants. Ask yourself if the child voice is what you want to follow this time. What has following this voice gotten you in the past? Recall situations when you didn't plan or commit. What have you done in those situations? Have you been able to eat healthy food in reasonable amounts or have you overeaten? What's your track record?

168.

A thought diet is a truly transformational diet. It involves giving up certain kinds of thoughts about food, such as "Hmm, what would *taste yummy* right now?" It stops us from romanticizing food, which is crucial, because the moment we start fantasizing about how a food would look, smell, or taste, we create desire and desires demand fulfillment.

169.

For many of us, the pattern of indulging our food fantasies has become our default position. Once the fantasizing gains momentum, though, it's like trying to stop an oncoming freight train. There's almost no way to stop it once it gets rolling. Planning can help you jump-start pragmatic thinking and put the kibosh on these kinds of romantic food thoughts. If you stop thinking about food romantically, your relationship with it will change and so will your weight. *You can change your romantic relationship with food by learning not to think about it or to think about it pragmatically.* If you have a food plan and you find yourself thinking about food that's not on it, turn away from those thoughts. If you have a set menu for the day, there's no room for food fantasies, only for functional thoughts like "Okay, these are the two options and this one makes sense." This way of thinking about food frees up your mind for other pursuits. It also becomes easier the more you do it. When you find yourself starting to fantasize about a food, stick to your thought diet and focus on something else.

170.

When you start eating more nutritious food, cutting out junk, and letting yourself get hungry before you eat, you discover that *healthy food starts tasting so much better!* That's because your taste buds become re-accustomed to the flavors of the nutritious, whole foods the body was designed to eat. By allowing yourself to get hungry before you eat, you help your taste buds along in this process. Because healthy foods are satisfying and don't cause you to overeat the way pleasure foods do, you tend to eat them in moderate amounts. As you begin to retrain your taste buds, jot down a few thoughts about what it's like to eat healthy foods now that you are restricting pleasure foods. What did the carrot or orange taste like? How did you feel afterwards? Were you satisfied or did the healthy foods leave you wanting more?

171.

When you're identified with the Dreamer, the hope of being admired motivates you to diet, and keeps you on a diet by spinning fantasies about the kind of life you'll lead, the clothes you'll wear, and the partner you'll attract in your new, svelte body. If you fall off the wagon, look out! The Critic will be right there, calling you every name in the book for going off your diet. The Critic uses moral judgments about food and browbeating to keep you on a diet, while the Dreamer motivates you with the lure of desire fulfillment. (The Child, of course, tries to keep you eating pleasure food the whole time.) Your true self encourages you to bring your body back into balance by prioritizing health, freedom, and happiness. Your true self moves you to change your diet permanently rather than go on another diet temporarily.

172.

If you're aligned with your true self, you see the whole picture about what food can and cannot offer you—and what a thinner body can and cannot offer you—rather than deluding yourself about how great life will be after you lose weight. You live in the present moment and remember that your ultimate goal is freedom from the conditioning that has kept you suffering.

173.

To the ego, exercise, like dieting, is a means to an end, a strategy to get a sexy body that it thinks will bring admiration and success. Other than that, the ego has no use for it. Just as it's perfectly happy to go on unhealthy crash diets to get a sleek body, the ego has no compunction about jumping into a punishing exercise regime rather than building up to it slowly with health in mind. Your true self values nourishment and self-care, and delights in the feeling of being alive. Noticing that your body's energy is waning, it sends a message urging you to rest or sleep. Seeing that your body would benefit from movement, it plants the idea of going for a walk. It actually enjoys the feeling of exertion and well-being that comes from moderate exercise.

174.

If yo-yoing has been your pattern, as your thinking comes into balance and your eating naturally follows, your weight might continue to swing for a while. Over time, though, the size of the swings will gradually diminish. For example, if your weight used to swing by 30 pounds, it may swing by 20 pounds, then by 10, then by 5, then by just 1 or 2 pounds. Keep in mind that most people can't go from swinging by 20 or 30 pounds to 1 or 2 in a short period.

175.

If you're still yo-yoing, you may think you're not progressing, not healing. But healing is a process, not an instantaneous fix. The key is patience. Don't torment yourself if you find that your weight continues to go up and down for a while. It's natural. Don't get discouraged if you're finding it difficult to put these new habits into practice. Looking for fulfillment and relief by way of pleasure food has been your pattern. Repeating it has strengthened and reinforced it, so it's not surprising that it takes time and practice before you're able to make a new choice.

176.

Have you backslid? If so, it's to be expected—it's a natural part of the process. It certainly *doesn't* mean that you've fallen off the wagon and won't heal. Healing may not happen on the ego's timetable, so remember to be gentle with yourself and let it be okay to make mistakes. Permanently healing eating issues is a maturation process. There's a part of you that hasn't grown up yet. Once it begins to mature, there's no turning back. When sixth graders write book reports, they don't have to strain to remember how to form the letter "f." That knowledge already lives in them. It's the same way with the Five Steps. Once you've learned them, you may backslide occasionally, but that knowledge will stay with you.

177.

Now that you're coming out of denial, seeing the truth, and changing your old habits, you can never go unconscious again. Following the Five Steps develops that part of you that never grew up in relationship to food; you become the wise parent and align with your true self. When you've dieted in the past, the diet book took on the role of the wise parent. But after the diet, if you hadn't changed the way you thought about food, your relationship with it never had a chance to mature and you've been stuck repeating the same pattern ever since. Now is your chance to change it for good.

178.

If you have a love affair with food, it means that you are using food to satisfy needs that it was never designed to fulfill. This is a happiness issue. When you're not feeling happy, it's natural to go after pleasure food, hoping to trade your current experience for one you think you will like better. Wise living, the fourth step, is an opportunity to explore how the way you're living and expressing yourself might be keeping your natural happiness from you. It's a chance to learn why you feel you need to look for pleasure from food.

179.

If you're fighting with people, castigating yourself, or afraid to ask for what you want or to say "no," the ego has you locked up, and will keep you racing to the fridge faster than a roadrunner on steroids. Fighting strengthens the ego: peace aligns you with your heart. If you want to stop eating your feelings, reducing your reactivity to others can be a great help. Improving your communication skills can help you accomplish this and at the same time create adaptive, positive relationships.

180.

Everyone wants to be happy, but not everyone tries to get happy through food. Ask yourself what seems to be missing for you? How are your relationships? Is your life the way you want it to be? Do you wake up excited to see what a new day will bring? If you're not happy because the structures in your life don't suit you and your relationships aren't harmonious, it's going to be hard to change your eating habits because you're using eating as a crutch to manage your unhappy life. Instead, why not take steps to change your life by beginning to arrange it to support your happiness? Once you start to make changes in your life to support your happiness and see through any conditioning that's been blocking your joy, you align with your true self. You learn a new way of being, living, and expressing yourself from your heart. This pays dividends in all areas of your life.

181.

When we make choices from our head, they're often fear-based, arising from a defensive posture that mistrusts life. Following our head means following the ego's strategy, which often involves finding ways to keep a scary, imagined future—that we have zero evidence will ever manifest—from showing up on our doorstep and devouring us along with whatever semblance of a life we've managed to create. Living from the heart means getting quiet and following a subtle, intuitive knowing that moves you to do what you love and what you're good at. It means asking, "What would I really love to do? What sounds like fun?" and then arranging your life accordingly.

182.

The Child goes after pleasure following ego-based desires. These are all trumped up, don't deliver, and ultimately lead to suffering. Instead, I'm recommending that you live from your heart, align with your true self, and move toward what truly feels good and is fun for you. Remember what it felt like to be very young, delighting in life and in new and wondrous experiences. Learn how to live this way again by asking yourself, "What makes my heart sing? What do I enjoy and get excited about doing?" Then follow the insights and impulses that arise. You're meant to be happy in this life! Finding a fulfilling life purpose is learning how to live so life feels like an adventure. It's turning work into play.

183.

All people have to do things they don't want to do, but no one has to do work they don't like. In order to stop wearing a path to the fridge, connect with a life purpose that actually engages you and feels fulfilling, something that you love and are good at. When you're so excited that you can't wait to start a task, food becomes less interesting and sexy. You're in the flow, and no ego pleasure can compete with that high. From that place, food is simply fuel. It tastes good and you enjoy it, but you're so engaged in what you're doing that you can forget to eat, and only a gnawing stomach reminds you to stop and take a break.

184.

Happiness is something to be noticed, not attained. It's always present, if you take the time to notice it. Happiness is right here, right now and can never be attained in the future. Because our culture tells us that happiness is something to be attained rather than something to be noticed, we've become a society of doers. We *do* rather than *be* because we've been taught that doing will get us what we need in order to have a meaningful and happy life. Once we've gathered the external trappings of a successful life, we think we'll be happy. When we're too focused on doing, we miss out on our natural happiness. In addition, because we do too much and don't value feeding our souls enough—going within, resting, being quiet, listening, and meditating—many of us are perpetually stressed out. Does this fit for you?

185.

Ask yourself, "Is there a part of me that feels happy and at peace in this moment?" How connected do you feel with it? That is your true self. The more you rest in that part of you that is always content, the less identified you are with the ego, and the less you will look to things outside of yourself for happiness. If you aren't happy, it's because you're telling yourself an unhappy story, you're doing too many things, or you've made choices that are not aligned with what you love to do. Your mind can cause you to be unhappy because minds are, by their very nature, negative. For example, your mind could be telling you that what you're doing isn't meaningful or that you're not doing it well enough. So, it's possible to be living a life aligned with your life purpose but still not be happy because your negative mind saps the joy out of it. The mind declares, "This is how things should be and how you should be...but you're not. You're not doing it right."

186.

In our culture, we associate eating with celebration and parties, so when we think our lives lack enjoyment we try to create fun through food. The happier we are, the less likely we are to create a painful, out-of-line party with food. If we're are aligned with a fulfilling life purpose and we let ourselves rest more, ease up on ourselves, and allow ourselves time to just be, then our whole life feels more like a party, and we don't feel the need to create one with food.

187.

Your true self allows what is unfolding in life, intuits what is true in the moment, and moves in that direction. The ego has an agenda and pushes until it gets what it wants. Pushing your way through life blocks happiness. Have you noticed? It's such hard work! For example, the ego might push you to work at a job that you don't like out of fear. "You won't be able to pay your bills if you leave this job," it says. "Wait and see. If you leave it, you'll be living on the street." Pushing yourself, even when you're doing what you love, will cause you to become out of balance. Do you have a habit of pushing, pushing, pushing until you either exhaust yourself or get stressed out? Notice where that line is and take a break, even a short one, when you hit it.

188.

When we push ourselves beyond what we want to do, we're apt to try to make it up to ourselves through food. Grown-ups unwittingly introduced us to this habit by offering treats to us as kids when we cleaned our rooms or got a shot. Now, we offer treats to ourselves when we push beyond what we really want to do. When the joy goes out of what you're doing, stop, even if it's just for a short time, and pick it up later. If you are working at a job you dislike, don't just keep doing it. Tell yourself the truth about it. Try to find ways to be able to do what you want to do instead. Take steps to move in that direction rather than organizing your life to avoid what the ego fears.

189.

Just because thoughts and feelings enter our awareness doesn't mean we have to act on them—we can just *notice* them. Being aware of thoughts and feelings rather than merging with them and acting on them is a huge leap forward in our evolution, not to mention our ability to make peace with eating, weight, and our bodies.

190.

If you stop turning to food for comfort, you need to replace that relationship with something else. That something else is your own true self. You connect with it when you spend time doing your "9's" and "10's" and take time to feed your soul. Make it a point into move into the thought-free state as often as you can. Just ask yourself, "Is it okay if I stop thinking for a few moments?" See what that is like. Each of spends time in the thought-free state every day. We just don't know it. The thought-free state is that instant when you're looking at gorgeous sunset and your mind stops.

191.

Any time our attention is on sensation—what we are seeing, hearing, touching, smelling, or tasting—and we're not caught up in thoughts or feelings we're in the thought-free state. In these moments, we dive between our thoughts and align with our true self.

192.

Today see if you can rest in the thought-free state when you're waiting in line, walking to your car, or even folding your clothes. All you have to do is notice that you're thinking and ask yourself, "Where's the quiet?" You're always being fed from your deepest self, your true self. Acknowledging that and choosing to make the time to stop and experience it helps you heal and grow.

193.

The next time an unpleasant emotion arises, notice it, allow it to be, and then ask to receive insights and healing. *Noticing moves you out of thought.* Ultimately, freedom from any eating issue is about becoming more established in your heart. To do this, make the time to be quiet sometimes, and choose not to be in a lifestyle that's so busy and stressful that you're constantly getting lost in thoughts, emotions, and doing. Moving out of thought helps you weaken your cravings by strengthening your connection to your true self. The more you practice, the easier it will become.

194.

When you're being attacked, it's natural to want to attack back. This only creates an argument. Instead, begin by acknowledging the other person's perspective and empathizing with them. Here are four words that immediately diffuse a charged situation and keep me from reaching for food. If someone is upset with you, try responding with, "I can see that." By saying, "I can see that," we acknowledge the other person's perspective, they feel heard, and it's easier for them to move back into their own heart. When you speak to other people, try to see where they're coming from, to imagine how you would feel if you were in their shoes. Ultimately, all acts of hostility and abuse arise from a hurt place in the perpetrator.

195.

Aggressive acts are actually cries for love. When people are acting out of the ego, acknowledge that and know that it's not who they really are. Remember how awful it feels to be so contracted and have compassion for their suffering. Remember, when someone is angry, they're coming from the ego, so try not to get hooked or escalate the situation.

196.

There is no such thing as a nice ego. Whether it's ours or someone else's, the ego is mean and ruthless. Some egos can put on a nice face to get what they want, but they're never purely altruistic. When people are aligned with their ego and acting out its nastiness, it's natural to move into the same negative state. We're conditioned to take others' negative behavior personally and react by attacking, defending ourselves, or stuffing down our feelings. These responses keep us aligned with our own egos. Moving away from someone else's ego that wants to fight is far from easy. Your ego is also trying to push, dare, and shame you into the fray. If you have the presence not to fight, all the better, because a battle between egos is one you can never win.The best response to someone's negative behavior is to not react at all, and stay aligned with your true self instead. That requires only one thing: that you realize that the other person is in the ego and that egos egg other egos on. Once you understand that, you can choose to step back, notice what's happening, and *not take the bait!*

197.

Not taking the bait is a huge evolutionary step. A sage once said, "It is easy to be enlightened in heaven." Well, it's not as easy to be enlightened in the hell created by a bully or someone who's taking his or her foul mood out on you, but it's well within your power.If you're able to notice when conditioning has been triggered, either yours or someone else's, you can learn to sidestep your emotional-eating response. Miracle of miracles, you can even catch an emotion before it's been created!

199.

When people are criticizing you, it's just their Critic talking—not who they are. Although there may be a sliver of truth in what they're saying (that is what hooks you), because they're speaking from conditioning, you know that their words can't contain the whole truth. When people criticize, judge, attack, or blame, in that moment, they believe their conditioning and they're suffering. The best relationship you can have to them is one of compassion. Being able to respond with compassion when people are attacking us only requires being able to see the truth—that their behavior doesn't reflect who they really are. It's just their conditioning talking. If you can be present enough to recognize conditioning instantly when anger is coming at you, you won't have time to take it personally, and there will be no upset.

200.

You already know how hard it can be to regroup once you're upset, so the next time someone criticizes you, try saying to yourself, "That's just conditioning." Your noticing it will preempt your impulse to take it personally. Then, no negative belief has a chance to arise and subsequently create messy negative emotions. Whether conditioning is coming at you from the inside or the outside, the approach is the same. Notice it right away, label it as conditioning, and don't buy into it. That way, you can sidestep both the emotion and the emotional-eating response.

201.

From an early age, many of us created emotional connections with sweet, salty, or fatty foods, using them to medicate ourselves when we were afraid, angry, or sad. Now, as adults, rather than uncovering the painful beliefs that underlie those emotions and using inquiry to dissolve them, or expressing what is appropriate to others in the moment, we stuff down our feelings with food. Eating might delay and blunt our reactions, but when we stuff our feelings with food instead of dealing with them, we may end up beating ourselves up or taking out our upset on those around us in passive-aggressive ways.

202.

In a confrontational situation, your ego will urge you to settle the score by attacking the other person. Instead, try to find a place to be alone or at least away from that person for a while.

203.

When an unpleasant emotion arises, notice that you're aware of the emotion, and acknowledge that, therefore, the emotion can't be you. You're not the anger or the hurt feeling. Dis-identifying with it in this way greatly diffuses it. Next, drop your story about the situation and focus on the body sensation associated with the emotion. Witness it, but don't feed it with more thoughts about how bad or wrong the other person is. Just experience the sensation. After some time, you may notice the sensation beginning to shift or dissipate. Don't impose any timetable on it. Just give the sensation the time and space it needs. Once an unpleasant feeling has dissipated, you have a choice: to let the other person know what's come up for you or to deal with the upset within yourself using inquiry. If you choose to speak to the other person, do your best to do it in a neutral, nonjudgmental way. Make factual observations and express the impact that the other person's behavior had on you without blaming.

204.

Speaking our truth is healing, diffuses conflict, and actually brings us closer to others, while speaking the ego's truth separates, inflames, and escalates conflict. We know we are speaking the ego's truth when we find ourselves blaming, name-calling, globalizing (using words like always and never), and judging. In speaking the ego's truth, we act out and defend our conditioning; in speaking our true self's truth, we take responsibility for it.

205.

By expressing impact, we're not asking the other person to change. Instead, our expression might take the form of asking for what we want in the future, e.g., "I'd appreciate it if....". This isn't the same thing as telling someone he or she has to change, which can sound judgmental. How we say things and where the words are coming from make all the difference.

206.

When you acknowledge your weaknesses or admit you're having trouble releasing something, you know it's coming from your heart because the ego doesn't admit to its failings. Once you've expressed yourself from your heart, if you're still having trouble moving on, asking the other person for an apology can help. You can simply say, "It would really make a difference to me to have an apology. If that's something you feel you could do, I think that would help me feel better." Apologies move both parties into their hearts.

207.

It takes a lot of practice and self-restraint not to attack and not to go for the pleasure food. If you tend to react immediately, changing this habit will require time, so be patient and gentle with yourself, just like you would be if you were teaching something new to a young child.

208.

Compulsive eating stems from repressing feelings—usually anger—and may require therapy to heal. Everyone has repressed emotions. It only becomes a problem when they cause us to hurt others or to become self-destructive. In our innocence, we eat compulsively because we think that distracting ourselves from unpleasant feelings is the best way to take care of ourselves. We're uncomfortable and use food to create an experience that we hope feels better. Instead, we end up eating self-destructively.

209.

If making art is your passion, you may not follow it because you're afraid that you won't be able to earn a living as an artist. Or if you aren't cut out for parenthood, you may end up having children because of conditioning that says you should. If you follow your conditioning instead of your heart, you may be living a life that doesn't fit for you. Unless you change that, you'll continue to feel unhappy, repress your feelings, and eat compulsively. To heal compulsive eating, find out what you've been repressing. Take a moment and ask yourself the following questions: What am I repressing? What am I angry about? Is there anything I'm not doing out of fear or habit? Is there anything I'm keeping myself from saying? How do I avoid asserting myself? What am I afraid of? Simply allow the answers to surface in their own time. Even if you discover an ego-based desire that you're not following, it's not healthy to repress it. If you choose to pursue a desire from the ego, don't fret because even going after egoic desires can lead to growth and evolution.

210.

Asking questions demonstrates your willingness to see the truth about how you've been living. How are you not living your truth? How are you not speaking your truth? By asking rather than thinking you already know the answers, you're humbly admitting that you don't know. You're surrendering to your own higher wisdom and are asking to be shown the areas of your life that you are in denial about. After you find out what you've been repressing, take action. Do or say what you've been avoiding and set the intention to stop repressing your emotions in the future.

211.

Healing is one part excavation and one part relearning and retooling. If you want to stop stuffing yourself with Oreos at the next sign of stress, you've got to change how you're living, how you're responding to life's little (and not-so-little) hiccups. In this way, you will to learn to break the habit of repressing in the first place!

212.

Another way to stop repressing is to become more assertive. If you feel that you're not entitled say "no" or stand up for yourself, you will probably get angry and either repress or feed your feelings. When this happens, you're likely to eat at the same time that you're having an angry conversation in your head. You heal this pattern by expressing what you need to express from your heart and attending to the emotional issue that's come up rather than feeding it with food and more thoughts. You might be afraid that people won't like you or that your spouse will leave you if you start speaking your truth, saying "no" when you mean "no," or asking for what you want. When those kinds of fearful beliefs come up, record them in your journal and test them by taking them to inquiry. Then, ask yourself, "What's the worst thing that could happen if I express myself?"

213.

If you're angry or resentful about the way your life is set up, you may need to make some changes. Stop doing things that you don't want to do, or at least take steps in that direction. Even though you may feel locked into your life, you don't have to spend most of your time doing things you don't want to do. To become empowered and stop repressing and eating your feelings, redirect your life so that you're doing what you love. Unless you acknowledge that you're *choosing* how you spend your time, you'll feel victimized, angry, and resentful, and be much more likely to eat emotionally. Eliminate as many unpleasant tasks and activities as possible from your life, so that you can be happy.

214.

Often, we get going in the wrong direction because our minds or other people's minds tell us we *have* to do this or that to attain a certain standard of living or to survive. But if you're doing what you enjoy, you won't need to get happiness from things or from food.There are two kinds of happiness, the ego's version and real happiness, and they look very different. In exchange for doing things you hate, the ego offers you a nice car or house or a big piece of chocolate cake as a reward so that you can feel good about yourself. But you don't have to get happiness from feeling good about yourself on an egoic level. When you're being true to yourself, you feel good because you genuinely like what you're doing. Then, feeling good isn't conditional. You won't need to be famous, beautiful, sexy, or rich to feel good about yourself. If living your heart's truth or following your passions doesn't generate the money, success, or admiration the ego desires, then so be it. It takes courage to live simply, doing what you love instead of having all the niceties that other people think you need, but it can allow you to experience real happiness.

215.

Negative self-talk creates low self-esteem. When we tell ourselves that we're lazy or lack self-control or anything else that's negative, we're acting as the ego's mouthpiece. In those moments, we rattle off negative self-talk as if it's actually true. Thanks to countless repetitions and reinforcement, we eventually come to accept this negative rap as a factual depiction of who we are, and we no longer question it. Negative self-talk is like a witch's incantation: It's mesmerizing. To break the spell, you need a powerful antidote: awareness. Set the intention to *notice the way you habitually talk to yourself.* When you notice yourself falling under a spell and a negative feeling is on the scene, ask, "What am I telling myself to make myself feel bad?" This interrupts the pattern. If a thought makes you feel bad, you can know that it's not true.

216.

Take any negative belief to inquiry and you discover that it never tells the whole truth. Just because you have a history of falling under a particular spell doesn't make it any less a lie. Once you see the lie, the spell is broken, and the negative self-talk no longer has any power over you. If those thoughts arise again, *either replace them with positive thoughts, question them using inquiry, or turn away from them altogether.*

217.

Eating to feel better actually adds to the problem of low self-esteem by causing you to feel less attractive and worse about yourself. It's a vicious circle: Eating the cookies brings a fleeting, nice taste in your mouth and momentary relief from a negative feeling, but then you berate yourself for not having any willpower and not losing weight. Not eating the cookies gives you a chance to:

See what you're saying to yourself that caused you to feel bad in the first place.

Use inquiry to become free of the negative belief that caused the negative feeling.

Remember, changing a deeply entrenched pattern can take time. Please be patient and tolerant with yourself as you chip away at your old habits. Can you choose to behave differently—just for today?

218.

Your true identity *is* happiness, balance, and peace. In other words, there is nothing good that you don't deserve. When you move outside of thought, you can intuit the intention of your true self for both you and every other human being: health, ease, freedom, and balance. And if that is your true self's intention, there can be no questions of deserving or not deserving. Worthiness is a given. The very idea that you don't deserve to be happy or thin comes from the Critic. When you understand this, you can immediately discount it. The Critic is a nasty piece of work, the aspect of the ego that generates all low self-esteem. So if you notice that you're feeling bad about yourself, you've bought into the Critic's rhetoric. See that for what it is, remember that the Critic is a liar, and ignore it. Noticing that the Critic is on the scene will shift you back into the Wise Witness. From there, you will naturally experience well-being, and the concept of deserving cannot arise. When you're aligned with the Wise Witness, there is no *you* left to deserve or not deserve. There is just a wondrous place of calm and joy and a melting back into a natural state of oneness. From there, the question "Do I deserve it?" is irrelevant.

219.

The perfection game was invented by the ego to keep us striving toward an imagined future that will bring everlasting happiness. The problem is that even if we achieve some of the goals that make up the perfection dream, life never feels as good as we hoped it would. It never feels completely satisfying. The ego uses perfection to keep itself employed. It coyly assumes that if we stay focused on striving and the future, we will forget to notice the happiness that's already available to us.

220.

Being happy for no reason is our birthright. Happiness is always available to us and when we're quiet, when we stop thinking, we experience it. The Critic thinks we need to have it all together to be happy, and the Dreamer imagines a future moment when we "arrive," when the years of work that we've done on ourselves finally pay off, and our dream of a "perfect me" comes true. According to the Critic, to get from our current, flawed "me" to the glorious realization of a "perfect me," we have to be vigilant, tyrannizing ourselves every time our humanness shows up. Everyone can heal their eating and weight issues, even if those issues took a lifetime to develop. It doesn't happen overnight, though. We progress, plateau, backslide, and then move forward again. You don't have to get everything right to heal, and you don't even have to get to someplace called "100% healed." It's just the ego that wants to be able to say, "I'm 100% healed!" or "Look how perfect my eating (or my body) is now." The salient question is whether your eating or weight are negatively impacting your health. If not, let it go. Why torment yourself? Ask yourself, "Is it okay for me to be human? Is it okay to be imperfect?"

221.

There's no such thing as a perfect person. Certain people appear to have it all together, but can we really know their experience? Can we know what their life feels like? Everyone's life has built-in challenges. Otherwise, how would we grow? Imagine how boring life would be without them. Can you learn to be tender with yourself even when you don't meet your own expectations? Knowing that life isn't easy, can you learn to be tolerant and loving toward yourself? If we're going to try to perfect something, why not try to perfect being kind inside? Why not try to perfect accepting yourself, especially when you let yourself down or don't meet your own expectations?

222.

Creating a wise relationship with your body means accepting your body just as it is and allowing change to happen from a place of tenderness, rather than forcing your body to change as a result of the Critic's loathing or the Dreamer's fantasizing. It may seem contradictory for me to suggest that you accept your body and at the same time decide to lose weight to improve your health. But to reject the reality of your current body size is to suffer, and it doesn't even help you lose weight! Both accepting your current size and changing your diet to achieve a healthier body are expressions of honoring and loving yourself.

Many diets actually reinforce the voices of the Critic and the Dreamer. The key is noticing where the impulse to change comes from. If it's a loving impulse, it's coming from the heart and supports a new, wiser relationship with the body that leads to healing. If it's an egoic impulse, it leads to suffering.

223.

Can you even imagine what it would feel like to accept your body right now? It's a radical idea that doesn't even occur to most women. But not only is it possible, it's the likely outcome of creating these new habits. So why not start right now? Close your eyes, take a deep breath, set the intention, and ask for help to be able to accept your body exactly as it is now, in this moment.

224.

According to Hindu philosophy, the notion "I am the body" lies at the root of all human suffering. When we believe that we are our body, we think that when it gets old, we're old, when it's fat and out of shape, we're fat and out of shape. We are spiritual beings having a human experience, not the other way around. Your body may be heavier than other bodies, but fat can never be *who you are.*

225.

This pressure to conform to cultural standards of beauty and thinness doesn't feel good. When you have negative beliefs about your body because you're listening to the Critic, and you decide that because your body isn't up to par, neither are you, you suffer. To begin to detach from the idea that you are your body, revisit the idea of your body as a car, ferrying you from point A to point B. It's merely at your service, helping you get around and experience life in the material world. Your job is to keep it clean, fueled, and maintained. When you use a car to get from place to place, you don't confuse it with yourself. You don't think you *are* the car, right? So why would you think that you are your body?Ask yourself, "Who is seeing this body?" The answer is, of course, "I am." If you're the one seeing this body, how could it be you? Whenever you notice that you're identified with your body, take a moment to remember the truth—it's just your earth-exploring vehicle—and snap out of it.

226.

The root of our desire to get pleasure from food is fear. If we inquire into the beliefs that underlie our stress, agitation, anger, and sadness, we discover the fear of loss. Negative emotions sap our energy and are the biggest triggers for eating for comfort and pleasure. The more you can allow your negative beliefs about food, your body, life, others, or yourself to dissolve, the fewer negative emotions you'll create, and the less you'll be moved to eat emotionally.

227.

If you've reached your ideal weight at some point in your life, did it make you happy? You attracted more attention and admiration, but did that translate into happiness? Did you worry about maintaining your weight? Were the partners you attracted the kind of people you wanted to be with? If you don't like your body, *the thought* "My body didn't look right is causing your pain, not your body's appearance. Without the thought, the body just does what it does—breathing, walking, sleeping, and there is no suffering. What is having a problem with my body's so-called imperfect size? None other than the ego of course! You have had the perfect body all along! You have always had the perfect body to learn and experience through. You don't have to wait to be happy until your ego blesses your image in the mirror. You can be happy right now. You know this is true because you've experienced moments of happiness, regardless of your body size. *You're happy when you experience life directly, without analyzing or judging it;* and you suffer when you believe thoughts that say you look bad.

228.

The desire to be thin, when it comes from wanting to be admired, causes suffering and creates an "us versus them" worldview. In wanting to be above the crowd, we isolate ourselves from other people and move away from love. The truth is: most other people don't really care how you look; they're too busy worrying about how *they* look. The only one keeping score is your pesky ego! Thankfully, we can step out of the Critic and the Dreamer and relate to our body from the Wise Witness. When we do that, it's easy to follow intuitions that move us toward health, moderation, and balance. The Wise Witness accepts our body being overweight and, at the same time, intends that we bring our body back to a healthy weight. The idea that a perfect body will make you happy is just a thought, a belief. If you've reached your ideal weight at some point in your life, did it make you happy? Perhaps you attracted more attention and admiration, but did that translate into happiness? Did you worry about maintaining your weight? Were the partners you attracted the kind of people you wanted to be with?

229.

The key to becoming free from the belief that you can only be happy if your body looks a certain way is to see it for what it is—a lie, or at best a partial truth. You do this by remembering the times you've been happy at a heavier weight and unhappy at a lighter weight. Then, you can begin to dis-identify with the body altogether, whatever its weight. That's true freedom.

230.

The myth of thinness is: If we achieve the body of our dreams, we'll live happily ever after. After all, models and movie stars seem to lead charmed lives. So it's natural to assume that if our bodies looked like theirs, our lives would be great, too. The media images of hyper-thin female bodies create an impossible standard for most women to attain. As a society, we're body obsessed. Unwittingly, we contribute to this obsession through our own behavior. To avoid that, the next time you see a friend, try to refrain from commenting on her appearance or weight and comment on her inner state instead. Our Critic has a vested interest in keeping us feeling bad about ourselves because if we're suffering, we're more likely to follow its plans. The ego loves its own cycle—striving, followed by success, followed by failure, followed by more striving, on and on until we die, having never reached our happily ever after.

231.

If you accept being overweight right now, what does that mean? Does it mean you'll slide into being fatter and fatter and never be thin again? Can you try to accept that your body weighs what it weighs right now? That doesn't mean that it won't ever weigh less, and it certainly doesn't mean that it will weigh this much for the rest of your life! If you're suffering over not having the perfect body, over not achieving the Dreamer's dream, ask yourself, "Is it worth the suffering? Does it really matter?" What would happen if you just let yourself be the way you are—just for now? What does your excess weight mean to you? It's important to look at what the extra weight means because *the meaning you're giving it is causing your suffering.* Who is the one who cares that you might not look as attractive carrying the extra weight, the ego or your true self? It's the ego, of course. Can you accept the ego's preference? Can you accept not liking your excess weight? Is it worth the suffering that resisting the way your body looks right now causes you? Really look at this because *suffering doesn't change anything.* Not liking your body doesn't change anything. It only causes you pain. For this reason, resistance is an irrational stance. If your body is this way, you might as well accept it. Why spend even one second evaluating it? It doesn't serve you.

232.

Trying to lose weight for health reasons, to look and feel better is one thing, but trying to create a perfect body is quite another. If you want a perfect body, it's important to ask yourself, "Is that where I want to put my energy? Is that what I want to focus on?" Striving for the perfect body takes a tremendous amount of time, energy, and money. Look at what celebrities go through to look the way they do. If that's what's important to you, go for it, but realize that there's a cost. That cost of pursuing the perfect body is all the attention you end up giving to your looks. Your life becomes all about appearances. You only have so much time and energy, so it's important to ask yourself, "Does looking perfect matter? How much does it matter?" Looking perfect matters an awful lot to the ego because it wants to be admired for being beautiful, disciplined, and special. But there's no happiness in it because being admired for physical beauty comes paired with the suffering of trying to hold on to it. Aging robs even the most exquisitely beautiful people of their looks.

233.

It can be hard to love people who look so perfect. In fact, they sometimes lack the poise, calm, and inner beauty that others who are less beautiful possess because they've focused so much on outer beauty. Inner beauty and alignment with your true self is what makes people want to be close to you. Think of all the people you know who aren't beautiful but are totally lovable. Isn't it true that you love them all the more for their imperfections? *Being at peace with how you look rather than obsessing over it* is actually much more attractive than outer beauty. It's one thing to care about the health of your body, but there's no fulfillment or happiness in caring so much about your appearance. Try putting your attention and energy into serving others, being present with them, loving and accepting them, and seeing their inner beauty. Once you do this, you'll forget about striving to achieve the perfect body and stop suffering because you haven't. You have only so much energy and so much time. Where will you put your attention—on the inner or the outer? The outer is a dead end.

234.

Most of us look in the mirror through the eyes of the Critic. As we look, we zero in on our problem areas: "Am I getting old? How do my thighs look? Is that a new wrinkle? Is my jawline sagging?" The Critic sees flaws and because all bodies are flawed in some way, mirrors are the Critic's perfect tool. Once the Critic identifies your flaws, it urges you to imagine how others will see you. Then it comes up with a plan to fix you, fueled by the Dreamer's fantasies about being admired and the wonderful life you could have if you looked the way it tells you that you should. If you're suffering over what you see in the mirror, in that moment, you're identifying with the ego. From the Wise Witness, we can forge a new relationship with the mirror by simply not looking too closely. That means doing what we need to do, like brushing our teeth or hair, and then moving on. It means looking in the mirror briefly and not scrutinizing, evaluating, judging, or imagining what other people are seeing. If you can step back and become aware of *that which is looking*, you align with the Wise Witness and connect with its compassion for the contracted part of you that's unhappy with what it's seeing.

235.

Once you become aware of your negative relationship with the image in the mirror and the suffering created by the harsh, rejecting, perhaps even violent way you've been scrutinizing it, you can choose to stop any negative self-talk and develop a kinder relationship with the image. Negative thoughts such as "I don't like it."; "I want to change it."; and "That's awful!" aren't us, they're our conditioning. The more we realize that the mirror brings out the Critic, the more we can work to develop a different relationship with the image by being very gentle with it. The Wise Witness knows that this two-dimensional representation of the body isn't you. Only when you look deeply into the eyes of the reflection do you get a taste of what you really are—radiant spaciousness, beyond name and form. When we're away from mirrors, it's easier to become more aligned with *what is looking out from our eyes* (our true self) than with *what our eyes see*. When we align with the Wise Witness, we experience ourselves looking rather than as objects being looked at. When we believe we're objects, it allows the Critic to rush in and judge us. If you want to stop suffering over how your body looks, avoiding long looks in the mirror can really help.

236.

The lesson we can learn from body-weight issues and aging is that our inner beauty—our authenticity and comfort in our own skin—is what makes us beautiful. When you look into your eyes for a long time, it helps you break through the illusion of identifying yourself with your body. The image, the appearance, is transitory. When we're at peace with that, other people relax and become very comfortable with us. We transmit ease and contentment when we're at peace with ourselves and how we look, and that allows others to be at peace, too.

237.

The perfect body is the one that's appearing in this moment, the one that's reflected back in the mirror. Can you let your body be the way that it is right now? The truth is, your body is the way it is in this moment. You can't change that fact. Whoops! It's too late anyway; the moment is already over. To reject this reality is to suffer. You can either be at this weight and accept it or be at this weight and suffer. Which will you choose: freedom and happiness or suffering? It's up to you. If you can accept your body for now, it leaves you free to move forward from a rational place of health and balance. Acceptance of your body in the moment does not mean your body will never change. But if you resist your body in the moment, if you hate it, you'll stay stuck for sure. "But wait," you may say. "How can I accept what I don't like? If I don't like this body, is it still possible to accept it?" Yes. You simply accept that your body is how it is right now. It may not be your preference, but if you can allow it, you will move out of resistance.

238.

If you can let it be okay that the ego doesn't like how your body looks right now, you are outside of the ego. You are noticing the resistance and accepting it. It may seem subtle, but there's a Gulf of Mexico between thinking *you are* the flawed body and noticing that the ego doesn't like how your body looks. As you separate your sense of self from your image of the body, you're more able to view the body as just your earth-exploring vehicle, not a statement of your worth. You don't have to take its weight personally. As you begin to dis-identify with your body, the body that appears in the mirror will seem to be no more yours than the mail carrier's. You call it yours, but perhaps it's only out on loan—so why not care for it as you might a favorite car and stop identifying with it? Think about the absurdity of wanting your body to look different than it does right now! It can't it's too late. The moment has already passed. Wish all you want, in this moment, the condition of your body is undeniably and irrevocably what it is. It couldn't be an ounce lighter or heavier nor a millimeter larger or smaller.

239.

Your body has nothing to do with you. Your role is to be grateful for its service and to care for it like you care for your car. Becoming free from body identification is like chopping down a tree. We swing the axe over and over again, chipping away at the seemingly impenetrable trunk. From all outer appearances, our efforts have little impact, but we keep swinging. Then, swinging the axe for the thousandth time, without warning, one unremarkable blow fells the mighty tree. In the same way, this apparently intractable issue can topple in a moment. Look at your body objectively. Pretend that it belongs to someone else and evaluate it factually, using neutral descriptors. Here are some examples of neutral body descriptions:

> This body is five feet, three inches tall.
> The hair is long, blond, and wavy.
> The skin is pale.
> The legs are muscular.
> The shoulders are broad.
> The fingers are long.

240.

Close your eyes and find the part of you that's struggled with eating, weight, and body-image issues for so long. See the suffering you've endured. Remember the times you've experienced self-loathing, castigation, and shame for being caught in the crossfire between the desire for pleasure food and the desire to be thin. Feel compassion for your suffering and honor your perseverance in looking for a way out. Honor the humility that has allowed you to open to a new perspective, one that runs counter to conventional wisdom. See how you've tried to create moderation and balance in your life, struggled to overcome weight and body-image issues, worked on yourself, tried different diets, read self-help books, and endured the negative comments of others and the Critic. Take a moment to honor yourself and feel grateful for your fortitude and perseverance while grappling with some of life's most difficult issues. Congratulate yourself for having the courage to move beyond your old patterns and try something new.

241.

True healing is not a magic pill. Appreciate yourself for having the patience to endure a process that has its own timing and *is not instantaneous*. Now that you've come this far, you're at the point of no return. If you've already been putting these new concepts into practice, you're probably beginning to taste the freedom awaiting you. But even if you aren't ready to put any of the steps into practice, just reading about this perspective has irrevocably altered your thinking. By learning this new perspective and practicing using these daily thoughts, you're moving toward a healthy, balanced relationship with food.

242.

Surrender is a gentle seeing of how we innocently caused our own misery, and by virtue of that seeing, ending our misery forever. Contrary to the predominant cultural messages, surrender is an act of maturity, courage, compassion, self-love, and acceptance that says, "I accept this moment exactly as it is." When we see the whole truth about food and our bodies relative to our misunderstandings and false projections, that's surrender. When we earnestly set the intention and ask for help in healing our relationship with food and our bodies, that's surrender. Surrender is an act of humility, an acknowledgement that how we've been seeing things and behaving hasn't been working and has been causing us to suffer.One day, without ceremony or fanfare, you'll realize that you can't remember the last time you had a worry about eating or your weight, that you can't remember the last time you paid attention to or suffered over a critical thought about your body, that these issues you thought you would take to your grave are finally healed.

Resources

- For information about *Skinny Thinking* Workshops, conference calls, individual sessions with Laura, the forum, podcasts, and to receive the free e-newsletter, go to www.SkinnyThinking.com. There you will be directed to the Skinny Thinking Community where you can meet other skinny thinkers.
- Also, please follow me on Twitter at http://twitter.com/SkinnyThinking and check out the Facebook fan page http://facebook.com/SkinnyThinking#!/SkinnyThinking?v=wall.
- National Institute of Whole Health (NIWH), established in 1977, is the pioneer of Whole Health Education®, a Harvard hospital–tested model of health education and behavioral engagement. This outstanding integrative training is provided through a unique e-learning video format. The curriculum includes evidence-based courses presented by nationally recognized health, nutrition, and medical experts, filmed at renowned Boston-area hospitals and medical schools. These courses integrate medical science with natural health care and holistic concepts. For more information, contact NIWH at 888-354-HEAL (4325) or at info@wholehealtheducation.org.

Recommended Reading

Robert Adams *Silence of the Heart*
Adyashanti *The Impact of Awakening: Excerpts from the Teachings of Adyashanti*
Byron Katie with Stephen Mitchell *A Thousand Names for Joy: Living in Harmony with the Way Things Are*
Loving What Is: Four Questions that Can Change Your Life
Gina Lake *Anatomy of Desire: How to Be Happy Even When You Don't Get What You Want*
Embracing the Now: Finding Peace and Happiness in What Is
Getting Free: How to Move Beyond Conditioning and Be Happy
Living in the Now: Reflections from Another Dimension About Being Happy in This One
Loving in the Moment
Radical Happiness: A Guide to Awakening
Return to Essence: How to Be in the Flow and Fulfill Your Life's Purpose
What About Now?: Reminders for Being in the Moment
Diana Schwarzbein and Nancy Deville *The Schwarzbein Principle: The Truth About Losing Weight, Being Healthy, and Feeling Younger*
Stuart Schwartz *The Great Undoing*
Dr. Bernie S. Siegel *365 Prescriptions for the Soul: Daily Messages of Inspiration, Hope, and Love*
Eckhart Tolle *The Power of Now: A Guide to Spiritual Enlightenment*

8493212R00139

Made in the USA
San Bernardino, CA
11 February 2014